MALICIOUS INTENT

MALICIOUS INTENT

Murder and the Perpetuation of Jim Crow Health Care

DAVID BARTON SMITH

VANDERBILT UNIVERSITY PRESS

NASHVILLE, TENNESSEE

Library of Congress Cataloging-in-Publication Data
Names: Smith, David Barton, author.
Title: Malicious intent : murder and the perpetuation of Jim Crow health
  care / David Barton Smith.
Description: Nashville, Tennessee : Vanderbilt University Press, [2023] |
  Includes bibliographical references and index.
Identifiers: LCCN 2023031033 (print) | LCCN 2023031034 (ebook) | ISBN
  9780826506139 (paperback) | ISBN 9780826506153 (epub) | ISBN
  9780826506160 (pdf)
Subjects: LCSH: Cowsert, Jean, 1925-1967. | Discrimination in medical
  care—Alabama—Mobile—History. | Discrimination in medical
care—United
  States—History. | African Americans—Medical
  care—Alabama—Mobile—History. | African Americans—Medical
  care—History. | Medical care—Alabama—Mobile—History. | Medical
  care—United States—History. | Racism against Black
  people—Alabama—Mobile—History. | Racism against Black
people—United
  States—History.
Classification: LCC RA448.5.B53 S65 2023 (print) | LCC RA448.5.B53
  (ebook) | DDC 362.1089/96076122—dc23/eng/20230710
LC record available at https://lccn.loc.gov/2023031033
LC ebook record available at https://lccn.loc.gov/2023031034

To Desmond, Isaiah, Liam, Cyrus, and Mya—
the next generation of dreamers.

CONTENTS

We face the suffering of human beings,
Ground into the gears of machines,
That crush the joy of nurturing life.
Pit pleas for help against privilege and price,
Create jungles of community,
With rage the only source of unity.
While we sleep fitfully in isolated routines,
May we soon awake to common dreams.

INTRODUCTION

THE HEADLINES IN MOBILE, ALABAMA'S local press at the end of January 1967 focused on the suspicious death of a prominent white physician. Found dead with a bullet in her chest on her front steps, it was quickly ruled an accident. Her life and death were soon lost even to local memory.

Beneath the surface, that death, was but one of many lost to memory in a struggle begun by nineteenth-century abolitionists. All these murders became unsolved cold cases. The doctor's death, however, marked an important watershed for medicine in the United States, answering its two most perplexing mysteries:

1. Why have race related disparities in death rates, once again documented during the COVID-19 pandemic, persisted since the beginning of our modern medical system a century ago?
2. Why has the United States persisted in contributing to those disparities as the only affluent democracy not assuring universal health care for its citizens?

Health care in the United States is the "ultimate cold case." It captures all that is unique about this nation—one whose utopian vision of democracy has kindled flames all over the world but has avoided confronting its own racial realities.

Most answers to these two questions blame "structural racism" but get vague in describing what it is. While the watershed Civil Rights Act of 1964 prohibited "racial discrimination," it never defined what that was. Current advocates of "antiracism" avoid confronting the "structural" part. They argue that it is just an easy excuse to do nothing. Most focus on "organizational culture" and all the conscious and unconscious biases that shape hiring, promotion, and treatment decisions.

This focus, however, flies in the face of everything we have learned about how health care works. All efforts to improve care—licensure, accreditation, and other credentialing of providers—focus first on developing the right structures.[1]

One concrete example of a major structural change is the desegregation of hospitals with the implementation of Medicare in 1966.[2] Medicare refused to make payment contracts with segregated hospitals that either did not serve Black citizens or served them in segregated settings. Title VI of the 1964 Civil Rights Act prohibited the use of any federal funds by any entities that racially discriminated. The requirement transformed the nation's hospitals from the most segregated public service institutions to the most integrated ones overnight. The most profound structural change affecting racial disparities since then, unfortunately, has been the result of court decisions that ended the threat of Title VI sanctions compounded by Medicare and Medicaid "reforms" that ended the ability of these two programs to serve as effective enforcers.

Structural racism in health care is easy to define. It asks, two obvious questions. First, how separate is the care different income and racial groups receive? If people of different races or incomes see the same providers in the same settings at the same times and are referred to the same places for other services, there is no structural problem. If they are to a degree segregated, one asks the second question—how equal is the care? That is, are the patients of different races or income groups served by providers with the same credentials and treated the same? It is the same two questions asked in the *Brown v. Board of Education* decision about public schools.

De facto segregation is, of course, harder to address than the segregation imposed by Jim Crow. Patterns of geographic and residential segregation and insurance status shape it. Most hospitals and physicians do not take responsibility for any of the segregation in medical care that results. Yet, the location of a hospital or practice determines the racial composition and insurance status of its patients. Providers have never been successfully prosecuted for "redlining" practice or hospital relocations. Except for emergency rooms, the legal system has never successfully prosecuted providers for instructing their clerical staff to refuse to schedule visits or admissions for those lacking acceptable insurance. Providers can defend such practices as a business necessity. Conscious and unconscious bias of individual physicians and other providers contribute, but the major contributors to disparities in treatment and outcomes are the structural ones.

White conscious and unconscious cultural biases created that structure. Public aid, care for the medically indigent, and other programs set up to help those struggling in poverty got defined as programs for Black people, even though most receiving help from such programs are white. This distorted belief contributes to the perpetual underfunding of these programs and a widening wealth gap between racial groups. Alabama's Constitution in 1901, for example, was designed to disenfranchise Black voters by imposing economic restrictions on eligibility (explicit exclusion by race was prohibited by the federal constitution).[3] Ironically, the provisions disenfranchised more white residents than Black, most voting for their own disenfranchisement.

Figure 1 portrays structural racism as a set of three nested cages

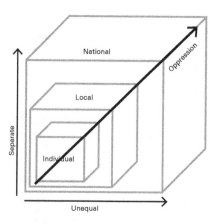

FIGURE 1. The structure of Jim Crow health care, 1920

restricting the effectiveness of the nation's health system. The outer cage restricts movement at the national policy level. The middle cage restricts the delivery of care at the local level. The inner cage restricts what individuals—patients and providers—can do to produce better outcomes. This book describes the construction of these cages and how we could end them. Most people take these cages for granted as just "the way things are."

Each cage has the same dimensions limiting the effectiveness of health care. The first two dimensions are familiar ones well covered by the history of civil rights and health services research literatures—racial separateness/segregation and inequality/disparity. Both have long shaped care in the United States. The 1954 *Brown v. Board of Education* Supreme Court decision concluded that separate education could never be equal and was thus unconstitutional. The Civil Rights Act of 1964 and the implementation of Medicare in 1966 came to the same conclusion for health care. The cages did not vanish. Both public schools and health care are still largely separate and unequal. The relationship between segregation and disparities are easy to measure and well understood—just ignored.

This book focuses on the third dimension—the forces that created these cages. They are a formidable combination of historical, cultural, political, legal, and economic pressures. In the past when these have begun to fail, fear, brute force, even murder did the job. The challenge is to reverse all these forces and move the "oppression arrow" to one of "resistance," making the cages collapse. That means supplying the economic incentives, legal reforms, and cultural change necessary to transform the two questions posed by this book into artifacts of the past.

I hope to flesh this story out for the general reader. Those preparing for careers in medicine and allied health are an ideal audience. Little in their preparation offers help in understanding these forces and how they answer US health care's two unsolved mysteries. I hope that this book will challenge them to ask more questions that had not occurred to them before. They need to step into this past if they are to help in repairing it.[4]

"Jim Crow" is a colloquial shorthand for the structure that shapes the way we organize and pay for care in the United States. I use it in lieu of "structural racism" because it is less accusatory of those that played no role in its creation and to acknowledge that there is always the hope that it is a fading artifact of our past. One would hope that the Jim Crow structure of health care has outlived the ideology of white supremacy that created it. Arguably, its imprint on health care now in this country is analogous to the QWERTY keyboard on mechanical typewriters, created in 1873 to prevent keys from sticking together. The QWERTY design has never changed even though the reason for it no longer exists. This is a commonly used example of what public policy analysts and historians call "historical institutionalism" or "path dependency." Once you travel in one direction, it is hard to turn around and go in another.[5] We take the inherited "structural racism" embedded in health care for granted. It is not consciously racist, just invisible.

President Obama, for example, used such an argument in justifying the approach chosen for organizing and financing health care under the Affordable Care Act of 2010. "Among many progressives the need to replace private insurance and for-profit health care with a single-payer system like Canada was an article of faith," Obama explains. "Had we been starting from scratch, I would have agreed with them."[6] For the alpha numeric keyboard on a computer, its persistence is no tragedy. Any theoretical advantage to changing the organization of keys would be more than outweighed by the millions of touch typists such a change would have driven insane. However, for the organization and financing of the health system of the United States, change is essential for preserving sanity.

Do we really want to perpetuate a Jim Crow health system? A brilliant idealistic physician asked that question at a key turning point in 1966. Her answer was no, and it led to her death, a cold case buried, just as the Jim Crow structure of our health system is. Unearthing her story is central to solving the mysteries posed in this book.

This book will explore what most leave out of historical accounts of the development of our modern health system, focusing on answering the two mysteries posed at the beginning of this preface. I have tried to keep the narrative simple adding endnotes for more complicated asides that capture more of the complexities and ironies. I will focus on concrete cases and the characters in them that I find fascinating. I have organized the book into three sections. They supply case examples of the three nested cages in Figure 1. Each digs into deeper layers, following the logic of an autopsy.

In the first section, I start with a brief description of the immediate events leading up to a talented physician's death, a teaser common in murder mysteries. I then supply a bird's eye view of how Jim Crow shaped the cage in which health care evolved in the United States. Finally, I "follow the money"—how Jim Crow shaped the development of the health insurance system that, in turn, reinforced the Jim Crow structure of care.

In the second section, I focus on a single community, Mobile, Alabama and the cage that evolved out its distinctive history. Mobile was never the focus of national civil rights attention. It never dominated national coverage about police brutality and Klan bombings like Birmingham, Alabama, which kept the national television audience glued to the nightly news in the 1960s. Nor did it ever grab national attention like Jackson, Mississippi did in the wake of the Klan assassinations of civil rights activists. None regarded it as a major seedbed for the civil rights struggle, as was the case with Montgomery and the bus boycott, Greensboro and the student sit-in movement, or Nashville and the Freedom Rides. In a two-volume compilation of national reporting on civil rights between 1941 and 1973, only the Mobile shipyard riot in 1943 that left about twenty Black ship workers injured gets a single sentence mention and, in 1963, the Mobile County School District was among those receiving federal funds against whom the Department of Health Education and Welfare brought desegregation suits.[7] Nor was Mobile noted as an initiator of change in the organization and financing of health care. It just adapted to the waves of change in medicine and health financing begun elsewhere. What Mobile does offer is a story that fits the complexity of the nation as a whole and the myriad of ways to stymie universal access to care and closing the racial divide. I focus first on the contribution of the old wounds. The port of Mobile exported cotton and imported enslaved persons. The last city of the Confederacy to surrender, the lost cause myth still resonates. Mobile's civil rights battles never matched the violence of other cities but in health care they were among the most protracted. Mobile's Jim Crow cage was solidly constructed.

The final layer focuses on how that national and local community history shaped the life and death of an individual physician. Dr. Jean Cowsert practiced in Mobile during a key transition in the implementation of the Medicare program that forced the desegregation of the nation's hospitals. Her death serves as the central "cold case" that acknowledges the courage and persistence of all those invisible volunteers that struggled to end racial disparities in death rates and in the assurance of universal care. I describe her childhood and medical preparation, her involvement in civil rights in Mobile and, finally, the circumstances surrounding her death.

In the wake of the deaths of more than one million citizens in the COVID-19 pandemic and the upsurge of nationwide protests sparked by revulsion to police racial violence, we have a rare chance. We can reverse the direction of the enforcement arrows in the nested Jim Crow cages. We can recover the memories of past choices and make better ones.

PART I

Race and Recovery of Memory

CHAPTER ONE

A Forgotten Death

A CLEAR SKY WITH A FULL MOON shone over the nursery and home at 4350 Cottage Hill Road in Mobile, Alabama, in the early morning hours of Sunday, January 29, 1967.[1] Concealed behind the plantings and shrubs of the nursery, a light gleamed from the kitchen window. Dr. Jean Cowsert shared this home with her mother Elsie Mae and stepfather, Fred Hayes. Jean moved in with them after she returned to set up a medical practice in Mobile. Cowsert shared her stepfather's love of flowers. They took pride in the varieties of camelias, Alabama's state flower, sometimes called the "The Rose of Winter," that they grew together. Mr. Hayes had been asleep for hours. Hard of hearing, he was unlikely to waken. She had admitted her mother to Providence Hospital earlier in the week for a heart problem.

Dr. Cowsert was writing a note at the kitchen table to one of the Catholic Sisters who served as administrator at Providence Hospital. She was proposing that all the members of the order that served at the hospital participate in a program of regular screening.[2] Such preventive services had yet to become a routine part of medical practice, but she took seriously her role as Chief of the hospital's medical staff.

A rock, hurled through the kitchen window, interrupted her. She had expected trouble, but she was not a person one could intimidate. She grabbed her .38 revolver and went out the front door to investigate.

Waking early the next morning, Fred Hayes followed his usual routine and went outside to pick up the Sunday *Mobile Register*. Jean lay crumpled by the front steps clad in pajamas and a blood-spattered bathrobe. Rushed to Providence Hospital's emergency room, she was pronounced dead on arrival.[3] A bullet had been fired into her chest. The nurse in the emergency room noticed that the religious medal given by the Sisters as a token of their appreciation of her work, had been ripped off its chain and her neck was bruised.[4]

The Mobile Police Department launched a brief investigation. Dr. Earl Wert, the City's coroner, oversaw figuring out the cause of death. He served as the pathologist at the Mobile Infirmary, considered the premier facility in the region, and was a well-respected member of Mobile's medical community. It was a modestly paid piecework assignment and one that had been previously filled by funeral directors.[5] The position had none of the forensic resources that are typically associated with city coroner's offices today, or, at least, television show portrayals of them. Her revolver, found by her side, appeared to be the weapon that fired the fatal shot. There were no witnesses or suspects. The wounds could have been self-inflicted, but Wert was troubled.[6] The detectives told him not to ask any more questions and wrap it up. A day later Wert concluded that the death was the result of a "self-inflicted accident."[7]

Few believed the death was self-inflected, either by accident or on purpose. Wert later acknowledged his doubts. Jean Cowsert's mother, however, didn't want any further investigation saying only that "enough bad things have happened."[8]

Records related to Jean Cowsert's death disappeared. The autopsy report, the record of the police investigation, the correspondence related to her activities, and any record of the FBI investigation of her death requested by federal officials no longer exist. A handful remain alive who remember her, and fewer ever understood the significance of what she had done. Unlike the violent deaths of John F. Kennedy, Malcolm X, Martin Luther King, and Robert Kennedy that surrounded her own, no one saw hers as a seminal event or ever wondered if things would have turned out differently had she lived. We should.

CHAPTER TWO

Jim Crow
America's
Health System

JEAN COWSERT WAS BORN on August 25, 1925, in Pensacola, Florida. She grew up in neighboring Mobile, a city that lived in the shadow of its antebellum past as a thriving port in the cotton and slave trades. Jean and the nation's health system grew up in a Jim Crow world. Its "cages" shaped her life and the health system she practiced within. Ignored in most accounts of the evolution of the nation's modern health system, her story "connects the dots" that explain the persistence of racial disparities and the failure to assure universal care.

The construction of America's health system began in the first two decades of the twentieth century. It was built within the "cages" constructed by Jim Crow. Those cages were shaped by influential proponents and events outside of health care that constrained its evolution. A broader partnership between Jim Crow and Progressive Era reforms shaped the organization and financing of health care. That partnership privatized control, deferring to the judgements of professional elites. Physicians, hospitals, and medical schools also grew in influence on a wave of scientific breakthroughs that produced a profound epidemiological transformation. Those successes came with baggage.

Jim Crow

The Supreme Court *Plessy* decision (*Plessy v. Ferguson*, 163 US 537 [1896]) ushered in the Jim Crow Era (1896–1954). It served as the foundation for the construction of the nation's modern health system. Homer Plessy, the plaintiff in the case, tried to challenge what had begun to happen across the South after the end of Reconstruction. A New Orleans "Octoroon" (seven-eighths white and one-eighth Black), Plessy was arrested for refusing to leave a "whites only" train car as required by an 1890 Louisiana state law. In a 9–1 decision, the US Supreme Court concluded that the state law requiring segregated accommodations did not violate the "equal protection" clause of the Fourteenth Amendment. Segregated accommodations did not imply unequal treatment. Only Justice John Marshall Harlan dissented, arguing that the US Constitution "is color-blind, and neither knows nor tolerates class among its citizens. In respect of civil rights, all citizens are equal before the law. The humblest is the peer of the most powerful. The law regards man as man and takes no account of his surroundings or of his color when his civil rights are guaranteed by the supreme law of the land" (*Plessy*, 163 US at 569 [Harlan, J., dissenting]).

Harlan's dissent reflected principles of equal treatment now shared by most health professionals. The *Plessy* decision, in contrast, legalized a caste system based on color. In the South, it spread to include public transportation, schools, housing, cemeteries, and newspaper notices of births, marriages, and deaths. Even the Bibles in courts were labeled either "White" or "Colored." In the North, more subtle restrictive housing laws produced segregated patterns of education, employment, and health care that would succeed in producing al-most as segregated a social order as in the South.[1] It took sixty years of legal maneuvering leading to the *Brown v. Board of Education*, 347 US 483 (1954) decision to begin to end the more visible symbols of Jim Crow, leaving most of the less visible structural ones untouched.[2]

Black people adapted to the harsh Jim Crow realities. One, who later sought work in hospitals in the North, recalled a childhood in the South:

> When I was growing up, Dr. Bailey on Main Street in Greenville (SC) was the family physician. There was a separate waiting room for Black people, and you had to wait till all the white patients had been seen before he would see the Black people. If the white patients kept com-ing in, you kept being pushed further and further back. Later, when a Black physician set up practice in Greenville, Black people flocked to him. I got a bad virus when I was a little kid and was admitted to the hospital. I got a private room on a white floor. My aunt did wash for a white physician and that gave me special pull. I felt extra spe-cial. I remember when I was a teen, I had to help my grand mom go for care at Greenville General. She had cancer. We had to wait in a horrible small room for Black patients in the basement. We'd get there at 9:00, and we often didn't return until 5:30. The local morti-cian provided the transportation to the hospital. The understanding was that the transportation was free, but he would get the body. It wasn't a bad experience. It was the way it was.[3]

"The way it was" meant the surrendering by Black people to white-imposed Jim Crow, quietly awaiting the hoped-for peaceful development of their separate churches, schools, businesses, and communities. The *Plessy* decision rubber stamped "the Atlanta Compromise" proposed a year before by influential Black leader and president of the Tuskegee Institute, Booker T. Washington in a speech before the Atlanta Exposition in 1895. Up until this point in the post Reconstruction era, there had been largely peaceful accommodation in the South to Black enfranchisement, representation in public office, and access to public parks and other public facilities.[4] Both the Black and white advocates of segregation hoped that it would allow for peaceful separate development. Instead, Jim Crow laws began a wave of terror against any imagined threats to white supremacy.[5] Mobs lynched 4,084 Black people in the South between 1870 and 1950.[6] Less than 1 percent of these lynching led to convictions. This reign of terror in most cases ended Black participation in elections, the criminal justice system, and all but the most menial employment. Federal legislation to prosecute lynching, despite the efforts of the NAACP and other groups, was blocked for more than a century, becoming a federal crime only in 2022.[7] The reign of terror did not just exact mob vengeance on individuals, it also targeted the independent development of black communities that the Atlanta Compromise was supposed to protect.

In Wilmington, North Carolina, as in other Southern communities, the violence first targeted the largest perceived threat: Black-white political accommodation. In 1898 a mob of more than two thousand white men overthrew the legitimately elected Fusionist party (a white and Black coalition government).[8] It marked an end to the desegregation of public services, Black enfranchisement, and equal protection under the law. The mob expelled Black and white Fusionist leaders from Wilmington with the help of a Gatling gun and Wilmington's light infantry. They set fire to Black businesses and killed as many as three hundred Black citizens. The leaders of the insurrection, rather than facing punishment, became US Senators and Representatives as well as occupying key posts in state and local government. No one was prosecuted for these crimes.

The violence against Black independent development peaked during the bloody "red summer" of 1919. Black and white returning veterans competing for jobs worsened tensions. Similar race riots or massacres erupted in at least three dozen communities.

The Tulsa Oklahoma Massacre in 1921 became the most notorious of many similar early twentieth-century events.[9] Greenwood in 1921, the Black business district of Tulsa, was known as the "Negro Wall Street." Booker T. Washington could point with pride to its existence. The seat of African American affluence in the Southwest, it included two newspapers, two movie theaters, and a business strip including fine Black owned businesses. A mob, triggered by false rumors and joined by US National Guard troops raked the area with machine-gun fire, bombed it by plane, and reduced it to ashes. The rioters murdered almost three hundred African Americans. Tulsa held no one legally accountable and buried memories of the event along with the bodies of its victims.[10]

White supporters and key Black leaders began their efforts to block this violence in the aftermath of a 1908 race riot in Springfield, Illinois.[11] It was a northern city, the state capital and final resting place of Abraham Lincoln. White mob violence could no longer be dismissed as just a Southern problem. A white mob of as many as 5,000 went on a three-day rampage in August, lynching two long-time respected Black residents, killing, burning, and looting. The only difference was that in this Northern city, police and National Guard troops tried to protect the Black community rather than joining the mob. The rampage left fifty-five Black homes and thirty-five businesses in ruins. Almost 2,000 Black people fled. Officials prosecuted only one perpetrator and only for a minor offense. The National Association for the Advancement of Colored People (NAACP) was founded the year after the Springfield race riot, on February 12,

1909, the centennial of Lincoln's birth.[12] Sixty people signed the call for its formation. Seven Black people signed, including W. E. B. Du Bois, Ida B. Wells-Barnett, and Mary Church Terrell. It was the beginning of a long struggle.

Progressive "Reforms"

Jim Crow and the Progressive Reform Era (1887–1921) overlapped. Despite the contrast between the violent brutality of Jim Crow and the positive contribution made by many progressive era reforms, they blurred together.[13] They were like the protagonist in Robert Lewis Stevenson's gothic horror novel *The Strange Case of Dr. Jekyll and Mr. Hyde*.[14] The progressive reform side of the character (Dr. Jekyll) argued that the "scientific" analysis of social problems produced reforms that helped everyone. Anti-trust measures, a graduated federal income tax, labor, food, drug, and civil service reforms have survived the test of time. Others tied to the Jim Crow side (Mr. Hyde) have not.

The progressive reform movement got its support from an emerging white professional class of political, religious, business, efficiency, and medical leaders. The support of private foundations with the wealth accumulated by railroad, steel, and oil magnates enhanced their influence. In medicine, Dr. Jekyll and Mr. Hyde blended reasonable reforms with the perpetuation of Jim Crow. Most who embraced the progressive vision of progress embraced an Anglo-Saxon vision of "manifest destiny" or white supremacy.[15] Critics argued that the statue of Theodore Roosevelt on horseback with a Black person and native American walking beneath him on foot at the front entrance of the Museum of Natural History in New York captured that vision. It graced the entrance of the museum for more than eighty years. The Museum removed it in 2021. The statue will be relocated to the Theodore Roosevelt Presidential Library in Medora, North Dakota (population 129), scheduled to open in 2026.[16]

In fairness, there were exceptions to this seeming calculated white indifference to the plight of Black citizens during Jim Crow. Two, Julius Rosenwald and Lunsford Richardson, played key roles in the story told in this book.

Julius Rosenwald was born in 1862 in Springfield, Illinois, one block away from the home of Abraham Lincoln and a few blocks from where the 1908 race riot began.[17] His father, Samuel, had arrived with nothing from Germany to the port of Baltimore in 1854. Like many newly arrived Jews in America at the time, he became an itinerant peddler. By the time of Julius's birth, Samuel had settled in Springfield. He owned a clothing store and a profitable side business selling uniforms to the Union Army. His son would create the Sears Roebuck mail order empire, the turn of the twentieth century equivalent of the twenty-first century's Amazon. The Julius Rosenwald Fund, endowed with the wealth of that empire and guided by Rosenwald, would invest its resources in addressing the damage of Jim Crow and the failure to assure universal education and health care for all citizens.[18] Rosenwald died in 1932 and the fund ceased to exist in 1948 when its assets were exhausted. Rosenwald had supplied matching funds used to create more than five thousand one- or two-room "Rosenwald Schools" across the South. He overcame the resistance of white school boards, using the lure of grant funds to insist on fair funding for Black education. He also gave a sense of ownership to local Black communities by insisting on contributions in terms of fund raising and sweat equity in their construction.

The Rosenwald Fund also focused in its lifetime on the development of strategies for assuring more fair access to health care. As noted in the next chapter, this included support for the Committee on the Cost of Medical Care (1927–1932) and later efforts to support two of its key staff members, Michael Davis and Rufus Rorem, who helped transform the organization and financing of health care. In addition, the Fund helped finance the construction of hospitals for Black people that would assure more fair access to care in the South.

Rosenwald also supported Black activism. The Fund awarded fellowships to a "Who's Who of Black America" in the 1930s and 1940s, including physicians Charles Drew and Theodore K. Lawless, poets Langston Hughes and Maya Angelou, and writers W. E. B. Du Bois and Ralph Ellison. Rosenwald funds also helped support the early efforts by the NAACP to challenge the *Plessy* decision that would later lead to the frontal assault in *Brown v. Board of Education* on the separate but equal lie.

Lunsford Richardson's life also fits into the story told in this book. Born on a farm near Selma, North Carolina in 1854, he moved to Greensboro after buying a drug store there around 1884. Mr. Richardson would experiment in the back of his store, creating patent remedies. He sold the store in 1898 and founded the Vicks Family Remedies Company. One of those remedies took off during the influenza pandemic of 1918. Vicks VapoRub was one of the few medicines that could provide at least some palliative relief for those suffering from the influenza virus. The company amassed a fortune in sales, but Lunsford Richardson died that same year, a victim of the pandemic that contributed to his company's fortune.

Lunsford Richardson offers a redeeming example of Southern civility in the face of a wave of white terror.[19] An elder in the First Presbyterian Church in Greensboro, he became loved in both Greensboro's white and Black communities. He regularly taught a Sunday School class at a Black church. As his grandson observed, he and the city's police chief, a man with a passion for violence against Black residents, were the only white persons that, for different reasons, felt free to walk at night through some of the rougher Black sections of the city.[20] As the *Greensboro Daily News* noted in an editorial at the time of Richardson's death, "he never passed anyone on the street, young or old, black or white, without a nod and a smile."

The family donated funds for a major renovation of the town's Black hospital, and, in appreciation, Black leaders named the facility the L. Richardson Memorial Hospital in his honor in 1923. For the next two decades Greensboro was the only community in the South where the Black hospital was more modern and better equipped than the white ones. A request during World War II by leading Black citizens in Greensboro led to the christening of a Liberty ship *SS Lunsford Richardson*. Greensboro's segregated hospitals would spark a battle that would end in the racial desegregation of all hospitals in the United States through the Medicare program in 1966.

On the other hand, there were those in the progressive movement who came close to the pure evil of the fictional Mr. Hyde in Stevenson's horror story. The eugenics movement fell into this category. Eugenics is the science of improving a human population by controlled breeding to increase the occurrence of desirable heritable characteristics. Sr. Francis Galton was a Victorian-era British proponent, as well as an advocate of social Darwinism and scientific racism.

Indeed, the United States, the birthplace of Jim Crow, played an influential role as the international proving ground for eugenic practices. Eugenics movement supporters in Europe followed genetic practices in the United States with envy. As one German admirer saw:

> The forceful and decisive North American does not consider the traditional moral code and does not consider the individual to implement what he thinks is right. After he recognizes the importance of heredity in determining mental and physical traits for the entire population, he does not hesitate to proceed from theoretical reflection to energetic practical action and to enact legislation which will lead to the ennoblement of the race.[21]

The United States served as the model to follow in the implementation of the racial hygiene movement in Germany. Anti-miscegenation laws criminalized interracial marriage in twenty-nine states in 1924. The Immigration Act that same year, designed "to preserve the ideal of US homogeneity," passed almost unanimously. It blocked immigration from Asia and set quotas to preserve the ethnic distribution of the US population as it existed in the 1890 Census. Most states had adopted involuntary sterilization laws and the Supreme Court ruled in *Buck v. Bell* 274 US 200 (1927) that compulsory sterilization of the unfit for the protection and health of the state did not violate the due process clause of the Fourteenth Amendment. Private philanthropic support for eugenic efforts flowed from the Rockefeller, Kellogg, and even the Rosenwald Foundation. Notable progressives and US presidents Theodore Roosevelt and Woodrow Wilson lent their support to the eugenics movement. In a presidential address Wilson claimed, "that the whole nation has awakened to and recognizes the extraordinary importance of the science of human heredity as well as its application to the ennoblement of the human family."[22] German participants in the eugenic movement lavished their praise on the American experiment and its success at eliminating "undesirables."[23] Adolf Hitler also praised them in *Mein Kampf* in 1924. Once in power, German public officials carefully studied how the Jim Crow system worked in the American South and modeled their own approach to the Jewish population in Germany after it.[24] Dr. Jekyll had completed his transformation into Mr. Hyde.

No president better embodied the Progressive-Jim Crow contradictions nor had more influence on the construction of the Jim Crow cages surrounding the nation's health system than Woodrow Wilson (1913–1921). Wilson is a case study of how life experiences could combine racism with progressivism.[25] Born in Staunton, Virginia, in 1856, one of Wilson's earliest memories was standing at the front gate of his father's parsonage and hearing the voice of a passerby announce in disgust that Abraham Lincoln had been chosen and that war was coming. His parents supported the Confederate cause. He

absorbed all the nostalgia for the "lost cause" narrative that romanticized slavery, portraying it as a gentle patrician affair—the Civil
War was all about states' rights and about undoing the Reconstruction Era misrule. That narrative is reflected in his book *A History of
the American People*. He describes Reconstruction as imposing on
the South the intolerable burden of governments "sustained by the
votes of ignorant Negroes" and took a sympathetic view of the rise
of the Klan in defense of the old order.[26]

> Almost by accident a way was found to succeed which led insensi-
> bly farther and farther afield into the ways of violence and outlawry.
> In May 1866, a little group of young men in the Tennessee village of
> Pulaski, finding time hanging heavy on their hands after the excite-
> ments of the battle, so lately abandoned, formed a secret club for the
> mere pleasure of association, for private amusement—for anything
> that might promise to break the monotony of the too quiet place.
> The chief object of the night-riding comrades became to silence or
> drive from the country the principal mischief makers of the Recon-
> struction regime, whether white or Black. The negroes were gen-
> erally easy enough to deal with: a thorough fright usually disposed
> them to make utter submission, resign their parts in affairs, leave
> the county,—do anything their ghostly visitors demanded. But white
> men were less tractable; and here and there even a negro ignored or
> defied them. The regulators would not always threaten and never
> executed their threats. The Klan backed its commands with violence
> when the need arose. Houses were surrounded in night and burned,
> and the residents shot as they fled. . . . The more ardent regulators
> made no nice discriminations. All Northern white men and women
> who came into the South to work with the negroes, though they
> were but schoolteachers, were in danger. Many of the teachers who
> worked among the negroes produced danger as deep as that of any
> political adventurer. The lessons they taught in their schools seemed

to be lessons of self-assertion against the whites: they seemed too often to train their pupils to be aggressive Republican politicians and mischief-makers between the races. . . . The politicians came for the most part like a predatory horde.[27]

Thomas Dixon Jr. transformed Wilson's florid white supremacy myth about the Klan into a best-selling novel, *The Klansman*. D. W. Griffith, an early film producer, snapped it up. His film version, retitled *The Birth of a Nation*, became the first movie ever shown in the White House, at Wilson's invitation. Wilson's *History of the American People* was cited in the film. It featured freed enslaved persons (white actors in blackface) as the villains and the Klan as the heroes. The movie, which the White House showing helped promote, stimulated the rebirth of the Klan. Wilson's sympathies for the Klan during Reconstruction, as reflected in his history and in the film, helped encourage an upsurge in white violence against Black victims during his administration. On Thanksgiving night 1915, a cross was burned atop Stone Mountain, Georgia. The Invisible Empire had been reborn.

Wilson presided over the resegregation of the nation's capital. Federal government employment of African Americans had been one of the few positive accomplishments of Reconstruction. Black workers accounted for 10 percent of federal employees and for the growth of a large middle class of Black homeowners concentrated in the Washington DC area where the opportunity for higher level federal jobs became possible. Wilson, however, allowed the southerners he appointed to re-segregate the Treasury, Post Office, Bureau of Engraving and Printing, the Navy, the Marine Hospital, and the War Department. His appointees blocked Black advancement in these branches.[28] They created separate offices, bathrooms, lunchrooms, for white and Black workers, dismissed Black supervisors, and ended opportunities for promotion to better paying jobs. When Black leader William Monroe Trotter and others met with Wilson to protest, Wilson argued angrily that "segregation is not humiliating, but a benefit, and ought to be regarded as such by you gentlemen."[29] For Wilson it was a matter of assuring efficiency in the executive branch by reducing the "friction" caused by integration. "We are not here as wards . . . We are not here looking for charity or help. We are here as full-fledged citizens," Trotter protested. "Your tone offends me," Wilson replied. The meeting was over.[30] The resegregation of these federal offices persisted for three decades. Racial integration, Wilson had argued during his administration, would just foster corruption and incompetence in the conduct of government and business.[31]

Even the Wilson Administration's symbolic ceremonial gestures consistently reflected the vision of white supremacy. In 1913, Wilson gave the keynote address at the fiftieth reunion of the Battle of Gettysburg. It included large attendance by surviving white Union and Confederate soldiers. He spoke, "We have found one another again as brothers and comrades in arms, enemies no longer, generous friends rather, our battles long past, the quarrel forgotten—except that we shall not forget the splendid valor."[32] No mention was made of slavery, no Black people were in attendance, and no mention of what Lincoln pledged in his own address at Gettysburg: "That we here highly resolve that these dead shall not have died in vain; that this nation shall have a new birth of freedom; and that this government of the people, by the people, for the people, shall not perish from the earth."[33]

Wilson had one last chance to set the record straight, at the dedication of the Lincoln Memorial on May 30, 1922. Too sick to attend, his seat was left empty, and he would die two years later. The ceremony, however, spoke for him. It was strictly segregated. Blacks were forcibly directed to the colored section by a Marine who reportedly said afterward, "that's the only way you can handle these dammed n . . . ."[34] The only Black person allowed to speak was Robert Russa Moton, the accommodationist successor to Booker T. Washington at the Tuskegee Institute, who had advised Wilson. The white organizers, however, concluded that his proposed speech was too radical. Moton had hoped to link Lincoln to the larger Black struggle for racial justice. The dedication of the Lincoln Memorial to that cause would have to wait and come with Marian Anderson's concert at the Memorial in 1939 and Martin Luther King's "I have a dream" speech at the civil rights march there in 1963.

No US president's ratings have fallen farther than Wilson's. Even as late as 1992, historians and the general public still ranked him among the half dozen greatest American presidents.[35] A Progressive leader, credited with many of the era's reforms, he got high marks during his administration. A graduate of Princeton in 1879, the thirteenth president of the university, governor of New Jersey, and twenty-eighth president of the United States, his alma mater named its School of Public and International Affairs in his honor. That naming honor at Princeton, however, faced growing criticism. In 2020, in a final acknowledgment of that criticism, the Board of Princeton University voted to have his name removed, because his "racist thinking and policies make him an inappropriate namesake for a school or college whose scholars, students, and alumni must stand against racism in all its forms."[36]

Impact of the Influenza Pandemic

Most identified with the progressive movement were impatient with the "inefficiencies" of representative democracy.[37] The Wilson administration response to the influenza pandemic during World War I added to broader public skepticism. Wilson failed to protect the civilian population and its armed services from what was, until COVID, the nation's most devastating pandemic. His moralistic focus on the conduct of "total war" made it hard to conduct a parallel one against the flu pandemic of 1918 or even to acknowledge its existence. Combatant nations on both sides exercised censorship of the press. Spain, a noncombatant, faced no such restriction and its press published stories on the flu there. Although the original source of the infection appears to be traced to army bases in the United States and the later outbreak in Spain was minor, the name "Spanish Flu" stuck. The unwillingness to admit to its existence would hinder stemming its spread.

National wartime hysteria made Philadelphia an epicenter of the pandemic: a case study in what not to do.[38] Despite warnings, a massive military parade promoting war bonds went ahead as planned. Public health preparation was nonexistent. The first Philadelphia cases appeared among sailors arriving at the Philadelphia Naval Yard from Boston in early September 1918. Philadelphia's Public Health Director, Wilmer Krasen, denied that any threat existed. He made no contingency plans, stockpiled no supplies, and did not even create a list of medical personnel who could be made available in case of emergency. Just as others, he feared that taking any steps might interfere with the war effort and reflect poorly on his patriotism. Not to be outdone, *The Philadelphia Evening Bulletin* assured its readers the influenza posed no danger and was old history.[39] Several infected sailors died the next day, but the Public Health Director insisted there was no cause for concern. The Philadelphia Board of Health endorsed Krasen's assessment.

No one moved to stop the Liberty Loan Parade on September 28. It was part of an effort to instill unquestioning support for the war. Philadelphia had pledged millions of dollars to help fund the war effort. The Liberty Loan Parade was key to this fund-raising effort. Canceling it would have been seen as traitorous. The largest parade in Philadelphia history went forward as scheduled. It included thousands of marching troops and hundreds of thousands of spectators crowded along its route. The patriotism of Philadelphians could not be questioned. Many paid for it with their lives.

Two days after the parade the incubation period for the influenza ended and the devastation began. More than 17,500 Philadelphians died in the first six months, 4,500 in a single week, and 837 in a single day, October 12, 1918.[40] Five-hundred bodies crowded the city morgue with capacity for only thirty-six corpses. Philadelphia victims less able to secure coffins were unceremoniously dumped into mass graves dug with steam shovels. On the streets of Philadelphia's poorer sections, the scenes were straight out of the European middle age plague years. Horse drawn carts paraded through the streets as priests joined police in collecting corpses left on the porches or sidewalks draped in blood-stained sheets. The bodies were piled up in the carts on top of each other with limbs protruding from the sheets.

Some of the memories of that period passed on in families. Frank Fitzpatrick, a reporter for the *Philadelphia Inquirer*, recalled such a haunted memory in his own family shared by his grandmother.[41] Her father and Fitzpatrick's great grandfather worked as a mortician during the influenza pandemic. He operated out of his Center City dwelling, a narrow row home. The corpses were all normally dressed and managed in the front room that served as his workplace. During the pandemic, the corpses overflowed into the parlor and then back into the dining room. The flu drowned victims, and many spent their last hours sitting in chairs, hoping that it would help them breathe. Some were not discovered dead until rigor mortis had set in. Trying to arrange them reclining for proper viewing required tying them down. She and her sister arrived home late one night after everyone else was in bed. They had to find their way through the darkened downstairs, holding their breath, tiptoeing past the corpses. The ropes loosened on the corpse tied to the dining room table and its upper portion sprung up to greet them. She was jumpy and easily frightened for the rest of her life. Fitzpatrick recently toured the house by the invitation of its current owner. His eyes closed walking through the dining room.

The psychology of total war would close Wilson's eyes as well. A month before the war's end, Germany was prepared to accept peace on any terms. Troopships sent to Europe with infected men could have been halted, not affecting the war's outcome, but were not. Army Chief of Staff, General Payton March, feared that halting the ships would boost German morale. Wilson did not overrule him to halt the senseless transports, even at the pleading of Cary Grayson, MD, his personal physician, and close advisor. Those ships became floating coffins in which infection spread rapidly.[42] Decks became slippery from the blood of hemorrhaging patients, tracked by healthy troops. The dead were unceremoniously dumped overboard at sea.

By the pandemic's end, a half million people in the United States would die. It would account for 40 percent of the deaths to US soldiers in World War I, almost matching the carnage on the battlefields. In keeping with this wartime censorship President Wilson never made a public statement acknowledging the impact of the pandemic on troops or on the civilian population. It signaled an end of the Progressive reform era and a growing skepticism about a government that would shape the search for solutions in assuring access to health care.

Wilson's view of democratic political dissent against the war as disloyalty outlasted his administration. J. Edgar Hoover, a young recruit to the Justice Department in 1917, made a lifetime career out of the distrust of political dissent. He assumed expanding responsibilities to arrest alleged foreign agents and radicals under the Espionage and Sedition Act and became in 1924 the first director of the Federal Bureau of Investigation.[43] His lengthy career would support the Jim Crow status quo. Toward its end this would lead him and his agency into the secret extralegal COINTELPRO initiative to undermine Black civil rights activists in the 1960s.

All of this fueled a backlash against the government that reinforced the private voluntary approach to regulating medicine. Private professional bodies assumed full control of medical licensure, hospital safety and medical training standards, licensing of physicians, and the standards to assure the safety of hospitals. It also, as will be described in the next chapter, resulted in the abandonment of governmental health insurance in favor of an elusive search for ways to assure universal care through fragmented private and voluntary approaches.[44]

Epidemiological Transformation

Between the flu pandemic of 1918 and the COVID one of 2020, an epidemiological transformation took place. Jean Cowsert's parents both came from families that included six children, some not surviving to adulthood. As the twentieth century progressed, graveyards ceased to bury as many children, and family size declined. For the first time in human history, the major causes of death shifted from infectious diseases to chronic ones more associated with aging. In 1900 the four leading causes of death were tuberculosis, pneumonia and influenza, gastrointestinal infections, and diseases of the heart.[45] In 2018 the four leading causes of death had shifted to: diseases of the heart, malignant neoplasm, chronic obstructive pulmonary disease, and cerebrovascular disease.[46] Life expectancy at birth climbed from 47.3 years to 78.7 years.[47] Improved public health, a higher standard of living, and medical advances all contributed.

What this transformation meant depended on who was telling the story. For some it meant less need to invest in public health. For hospitals and surgical specialists, it meant doing more procedures to correct the chronic conditions of aging, constructing gleaming hospital towers devoted to this, and, for a few talented surgeons, seven-figure incomes. For those concerned with ending racial disparities, however, it meant a harder hill to climb. Despite the epidemiological transformation, differences in Black as opposed to white death rates remained almost unchanged. Black infant mortality and age-adjusted differences in years of life lost before age 75 stagnated for a century at rates almost twice that of white populations.[48] Germs and viruses do not respect color lines. It is easier to make the argument that all races and classes receive help from the prevention of infectious diseases. "We're all in this together" was a common refrain long before the COVID-19 pandemic. Supplying vaccines to individuals is cheap and everyone benefits. Open heart surgery is expensive and benefits only the recipient. Some, usually those with more generous insurance coverage, ask "Why should I pay for treating 'those other people,' who smoke, drink, or eat too much and choose not to purchase health insurance or can't afford the elective surgery needed for treatment?" These attitudes reflect the stark racial differences in use of surgical advances to address the ravages of aging. White/Black disparities in such surgical rates have remained at 2:1, even after the elimination of such differences became a national health goal in the 1980s. In 2011, the Department of Health and Human Services, determined to close this gap, launched a "national action plan." It began a coordinated effort through financial incentives and greater public accountability to assure more racially fair access to such procedures. Five years later, white/Black differences in surgical rates for these procedures remained essentially unchanged.[49] Neither region, type of insurance, nor teaching status of the hospitals involved made any difference. The report found the need for renewed initiatives to improve health care equality, repeating the same conclusion that justified the launching of the action plan in the first place.

Celebration of the heralded "epidemiological transformation" of deaths from infectious diseases to the chronic ones of old age proved premature, even before the COVID-19 pandemic. Wars, social conflicts, shifting poverty, growing urbanization, climate change, and an anti-science backlash had already ended the earlier steep declines and threatened a rise in death rates.[50] The rising toll in the United

States of "deaths of despair" from suicide, alcoholism, and drug addiction among the white male rural working class preceded much of the current political fissures.[51]

Pandemics have always proved to be powerful agents of social change. The Black Death in the fourteenth century in Europe killed one third of the population. It strengthened the bargaining position of a shrunken population of surviving craftsmen and broke the hold of the Medieval caste system, making the Renaissance and trade expansion in the fifteenth and sixteenth centuries possible.[52] That, in turn, led to European colonization of the Americas, the slave trade to support it and the founding of the United States in 1776. The "epidemiological transformation" bookended between the nation's two major pandemics may in the end prove illusory. Perhaps in the wake of the deaths of more than one million citizens in the COVID-19 pandemic, we have a similar chance to remake the social order.

In the end, the Jim Crow era set in concrete the structure of the nation's health system. The progressive movement's medical reform efforts took for granted the separate and unequal nature of care and the disparities in health. The segregated organization of medical practice, hospital care, and medical training persisted despite the elimination of the laws and labels. In addition, the failures of the Wilson Administration in ending Jim Crow terrorism, obtaining a more permanent peace in the Great War, and addressing the influenza pandemic increased distrust in government. All the "actors" in these cages—organized medicine, hospitals, and medical schools—accommodated to these constraints. The health system, despite its accomplishments, did little to reduce racial disparities or assure universal access.

The Caged Transformation of Medicine

Jim Crow and the backlash against government expansion set the stage for the development of the nation's modern health system. The key actors in the drama—organized medicine, hospitals, and medical schools—evolved in ways that avoided direct public oversight. While they argued that this best served the public interest, it also served Jim Crow.

Organized Medicine

By 1910 "organized medicine" had ceased to be an oxymoron. The era when anyone could hang out a shingle as a medical practitioner was over. In 1860 that ease of entry into medicine resulted in 175 physicians per 100,000 population, higher than in any other country in the world.[53] Later declines in those ratios resulted from the creation of local, state, and national medical associations and their efforts to restrict entry and assure better income for their members. The number of active physicians in medical practice did not climb again to match the 1860 175 physician to 100,000 population until 2015.

The motives, as acknowledged by its leaders, were economic and the means for achieving them political.[54] Despite pronouncements about their altruistic concern for public safety, there was no attempt to make the case for public safety based on scientific evidence. The two major "sects" that competed with regular or allopathic medicine, the homeopaths and eclectics, advocated for more conservative interventions and natural healing and probably killed fewer people. Allopathy inherited the tradition of "heroic therapy" including bleeding and purging of patients. Its national organization, the American Medical Association (AMA) was founded in 1847. According to AMA spokespersons, its three major goals were to:

1. Establish state licensure laws to restrict entry and secure better economic conditions for its members,
2. The destruction of the proprietary schools of medicine and replacement with fewer non-profit ones requiring more extensive training and producing a much more limited supply of graduates.

3. The elimination of medical sects (eclectics, homeopaths etc.) as unwelcome and competitive forces in the profession.[55]

With the help of affiliated local and state associations, those goals were well on the way to being achieved by 1910. The Mobile County Medical Society and Alabama State Medical Association had served as key models for this national political transformation. Jean Cowsert would join these two bodies on her return to practice in Mobile in 1959. She did not fit in and her relationship with its leaders, as will be described in the last section of this book, was a strained one.

Efforts to set up an effective state board of medical examiners in Alabama showed the political power of well-organized local and state medical associations. Jerome Cochran, MD, a post–Civil War era Mobile physician was credited with being the "Father of Alabama public health." His real major accomplishment, however, was transforming the local and state medical associations into "a medical legislature having as its highest function the governmental direction of the medical profession of the state."[56] Cochran succeeded in this task by engineering a near physician majority in both houses of the state legislature in 1873. Later legislation, in effect, delegated the power of governmental bodies to the state and local medical associations. The Mobile County Medical Society would end up serving as a board of medical examiners deciding who would be licensed to practice. The AMA, encouraged by Alabama's example of success, pursued a similar national strategy.

State and county medical societies of the AMA functioned not just as quasi-governmental bodies but also as white-only social clubs. Black medical professionals and other ethnic groups were excluded. Even if granted licensure, this would limit access to hospital privileges, continuing medical education, and malpractice insurance coverage. Membership was also refused on "ethical" grounds. Any physician's practice that involved some form of discounted payments that might adversely affect other members economically was defined as "unethical." As described in the next chapter, this would create a major barrier to assuring universal access to care.

Physicians also had to accommodate to Jim Crow laws in the South and comparable informal expectations in the North. In the South, a physician could offer Black patients either separate times or separate waiting rooms and would guide them to the right inpatient accommodations. In the North, physicians would similarly admit patients to hospitals by race, respecting more informal understandings that would assure almost the same degree of segregation.

Hospitals

The Jim Crow cage that hospitals evolved within was more complex. Nineteenth-century hospitals were the last recourse of the medically indigent. Those that could afford it were cared for in a doctor's office or in their own home. Hospitals were either public or private charitable ventures. The public ones included the infectious disease hospitals, state psychiatric hospitals, alms houses, and poor farms. They served a public health protection and police function. The larger urban public hospitals increasingly also served a teaching function. Medical students and private physicians volunteered to supply care in exchange for the learning experience. Private hospitals were an even more diverse collection of facilities. They served the whim of their charitable funders, some making the admission decisions on who was "worthy" of their charity.

Hospitals followed all the Jim Crow proscriptions. Disproportionately, Black patients were served by the public hospitals and whites served by the private charitable facilities that were increasingly dependent on patients paying privately. In the South, separate hospitals or sections served blacks. "Negro only" facilities were sometimes "donated" to the Black community by white hospitals moving to more up to date accommodations. Montague Cobb, a Howard University medical school faculty member who led the hospital desegregation effort in the 1960s, referred to this practice as "old clothes for Sam," donating the shabbiest items to suitably appreciative Black communities.[57] For facilities that served both Black and white patients, a wing or a basement unit supplied the "colored" accommodations. A substandard separate building often supplied the Black ward accommodations. Surgical patients had to be transported, often in inclement weather, between these two structures. There was no "equal" in the separate accommodations.

Many smaller southern communities had hospitals that accommodated only white patients. Critically ill Black patients traveled long distances in search of an accepting facility. Since local ambulance services as well as cab services were white only, patients were transported in Black funeral home hearses. The understanding between the funeral home and the patient's family was that the service was free, but it would get the body back for burial, often soon.[58] In 1952, the Southern Conference Education Fund published a report, *The Untouchables: The Meaning of Segregation in Hospitals*, that documented a dozen cases, including some in the North where such racial exclusions had resulted in unnecessary deaths.[59]

Public hospitals and medical school facilities supplied care for the indigent. In the wake of the Great Migration of Blacks to northern cities, Chicago's Cook County, Philadelphia General and New York City's public hospital system became sought-after internship and residency sites for medical graduates. The availability of "teaching material" was the major lure. Quentin Young, MD, who interned at Cook County in the late 1940s, shared a common ambivalence about the experience.

On the medical side it was a premier training place. I got there just after World War II, and it was still riding on its prewar reputation as a training center. It was a very sought-after site. Yet the patient loads were ridiculous, you had limited support and your training came from the residents and by the seat of your pants. I think it trained a lot of people very well, but at what cost, one wonders.[60]

The debt to Black people in the education of white physicians included what could be learned from their corpses. In the pre-civil war South, the sale of the bodies of enslaved people to physicians and medical schools was common and consistent with the logic of viewing them as property. The improvement in rail transportation after the Civil War expanded the market to medical schools in the North. According to the account of Dr. D. C. Waite these were supplied to northern medical schools following a well-organized routine at the turn of the twentieth century.

> A gentleman now deceased who was a demonstrator and later a professor of anatomy at a New England medical school told me a few years ago that in the "eighties and nineties" he had an arrangement under which he received twice in each session a shipment of twelve bodies of southern Negroes. They came in barrels marked "turpentine" and consigned to a local hardware store that dealt in painting materials. The receipt of two large shipments of turpentine in the season of the year when little painting was done created no suspicion as to the real contents of the barrels.[61]

In 1933, Montague Cobb, MD, Howard Medical School professor of anatomy, who later became instrumental in efforts to desegregate hospital care, published a study showing some southern medical schools had for many years taught their students the fundamentals of human anatomy exclusively with Negro cadavers. One never to miss such ironies, Cobb observed "This led to the conclusion that our colleagues recognized in the Negro a perfection in human structure which they were unwilling to concede when that structure was animated by the vital spark."[62]

Hospitals were a major target of standardization by the medical profession, motivated by a mixture of concern over improvement and professional self-interest. Founded in 1913, the American College of Surgeons (ACS) focused on imposing higher standards on those permitted to do surgery and on the hospitals where such surgery was performed.[63] Hospitals, just as medical schools, had no agreed upon standards. As already noted, most were private charitable organizations shaped by the idiosyncrasies of their donors. Board members made the decisions about who of the "worthy poor" would be admitted for care. The alternative, for-profit operations, owned directly by the physicians doing the surgery with not even the illusion of independent goal scientific control of standards, would have undermined the professional credibility of surgeons. In both for profit and nonprofit settings, "fee splitting," the referring physician getting a part of the surgeon's fee, was routine. The referring physician could choose the surgeon, not on skill, but on who offered the largest kickback. While the ACS succeeded in ending the most blatant abuses, referral patterns continue to be the most sensitive, controversial, and least well understood issue in the organization and financing of care. Discriminatory referral abuses surrounded the events culminating in Jean Cowsert's death and persist as a major contributor to racial disparities in outcomes.

Membership in ACS was intended to offer coveted recognition of the skill and professionalism of the surgeon. The problem was that there was no way to objectively make such a determination, The record-keeping system on surgical performance in hospitals was nonexistent. The last thing members of the ACS wanted was a system of government oversight akin to what progressive reformers had imposed on the meatpacking and patent medicine industries.

The special elite professional status that had been the purpose of ACS's founding would be undermined. Loyal Davis, one of the ACS founders who wrote a flattering history of the ACS's accomplishments, was also Ronald Reagan's father-in-law and was influential in shaping Reagan's conservative approach to government regulation as President.[64] Instead, the ACS invented its own private voluntary system of controls to prevent the intrusion of government oversight. Hospitals were invited to voluntarily take part in an ACS survey and certification process. In 1918 the board met at a hotel in New York to decide the fate of the participating hospitals. Of the 692 hospitals that agreed to take part in these survey visits only eighty-nine met ACS' minimal standards.[65] ACS reported only the names of the eighty-nine. They burned the reports made of the others in the basement furnace of the New York hotel where they met.

Was the ACS minimum standard program successful? As an educational tool, certainly. Record-keeping improved and the effort helped curtail fee-splitting arrangements with surgeons. The ACS's standardization program survives, now as the Joint Commission, certifying hospitals for payment from many insurers including state and federal government ones. It also provides hospitals some protection from malpractice lawsuits. Many other health professional bodies have copied the model. The debate persists about the effectiveness of such private voluntary bodies in protecting the public as opposed to protecting the professional self-interests of its members.

The ACS minimum standard requirement for an organized medical staff, however, also fundamentally changed the relationship of physicians to hospitals. Instead of charitable volunteers, they became the key decision makers. They decided what patients could be admitted for treatment and which physicians would have what kind of admission and surgical privileges. Their self-interests, the interests of their patients and racial biases of these collegial key decision-making bodies all blurred together. The standards accelerated the transformation of hospitals from private charities serving the "deserving" poor (those not victims of sexually transmitted diseases, alcohol, or drug related illnesses or at least of the "right" racial, ethnic, or religious group) into those that could afford to pay for their hospital and surgeon's care. Hospital privileges, instead of being a voluntary charitable duty, became key to the economic survival of surgeons and other hospital specialty physicians.

The ACS hospital standardization program, however, left the Jim Crow realities of hospital care untouched. Few Black physicians gained privileges at these hospitals and most had to rely on white medical staff members to care for their patients when admitted. Black hospitals tried to build their own standard-setting organizations and some Black hospitals closed.[66] Residency and internship opportunities for Black physicians were limited to the few Black hospitals that offered such opportunities. Care became even more separate and unequal and few leaders in the hospital reform movement saw any problem with this.

Medical Schools

Two private foundations, Carnegie and Rockefeller, played influential roles in reforming medical education while reinforcing its Jim Crow infrastructure. With their support, progressives focused on standardizing medical education and reducing the glut of poorly trained practitioners. Many American schools at the turn of the twentieth century did not require any college education or even a high-school diploma for admission. Some were just commercial diploma mills relying on local practitioners as guest lecturers and supplying little scientific background or clinical practice experience. Seeking reform and to hasten their elimination, the AMA set up the Council of Medical Education (CME) in 1904. Since a CME report making recommendations on the standardization of medical education would have been interpreted as self-serving, they arranged for the like-minded director of the Carnegie Foundation to support an "independent" survey of medical schools. Abraham Flexner was recruited by the foundation to conduct a survey of the 155 medical schools in North America then in operation.[67] He had completed an undergraduate degree in the classics at Johns Hopkins, but his younger brother Simon had graduated from its medical school. Unqualified to produce a document that would transform medical education, he was aided and abetted by the CME efforts to restrict entry into the profession and by the financial support of private foundations. Flexner's scathing report added fuel to the fire that would eliminate half the medicals schools and half the number of graduates by 1920.[68] He argued for the need to standardize medical education along the model offered by Hopkins, and to place the licensure of medical school graduates under the oversight of like-minded state medical boards already well underway. Carnegie, Rockefeller, Rosenwald, and other private foundations helped stimulate this consolidation by funneling funds to schools supported by the Flexner Report recommendations.

Flexner's document, however influential, reads today as a sanctimonious, pretentious, unsupported collection of opinions. In his survey of Alabama's two medical schools, Birmingham Medical College, and the Medical Department of the University of Alabama in Mobile, he concluded that "it is clear that satisfactory medical education is not to be had in Alabama. Entrance standards are low; the schools are inadequately equipped; and they are without adequate financing, . . . neither Alabama or the rest of the south actually needs either school at this time."[69] Nevertheless, his recommendation that the University of Alabama Medical Department be moved to a medical school in Birmingham was soon implemented.

Flexner reserved his most critical and patronizing commentary for Black medical schools. Only Meharry and Howard seemed worth saving, "The other black medical schools are wasting small sums annually and sending out undisciplined men, whose lack of real training is covered up by the imposing M.D. degree."[70] All five of these schools closed soon afterward. (Flint, Medical College of Raleigh, the Medical Department of the University of West Tennessee, and the National Medical College of Louisville). The restrictions in access to medical education for Black students in the next twenty years after the release of the report took place while nine of the nation's largest foundations plowed a total of $150 million into a select few white medical schools to help implement the report's recommendations.[71]

Flexner's view of women in mainstream medicine, in contrast to Black doctors, seemed a model of reasonableness. He saw no need to preserve separate schools. Historically male schools could easily accommodate qualified women. (As the number of slots in medical schools for students shrank as Flexner recommended, however, the number of slots filled by females also shrank).

The notion that Black trainees could be accommodated by these same white medical schools just as white females does not seem to have occurred to Flexner: "The practice of the Negro doctor will be limited to his own race" and "the Negro must be educated not only for his own sake, but for ours. He is as far as the human eye can see, a permanent factor in the nation."[72] Flexner took for granted that the Negro doctor, segregated by education and practice would remain subservient to the white medical community and be best used as sanitarians rather than surgeons protecting the white community from infection and thus justifying separate support. He wrote, "The negro needs good schools—schools to which the more promising of the race can be sent to receive substantial training in which hygiene rather than surgery, for example, is strongly accentuated. If at the same time they can be imbued with a missionary spirit so that they will look upon their diploma as a commission to serve their people humbly and devotedly, they may play an important part in the sanitation and civilization of the whole nation. Their duty calls them away from the large cities to the village and plantation, upon which light has hardly begun to break."[73] Black physicians never tried a formal response to Flexner's report, but some must have muttered expletives.

The transformation of medical schools driven by Flexner's report, the support of private foundations, and then federal research funding achieved much. A correction began with the shift in the bulk of medical school funding toward clinical services resulting from the implementation of Medicare and Medicaid in 1966. The post-Flexner reform preoccupation with the research mission may have contributed to such racial scandals as the Tuskegee syphilis "experiment" where informed consent would never have been given for studying the effects of not treating the disease on poor rural Alabama Black patients.[74] Johns Hopkins Medical School, the model exemplar used in Flexner reforms, in 1951 took the cells of a poor Black woman without permission. The cells were reproduced, resulting in scientific breakthroughs she and her family never benefitted from.[75] Some called for rebalancing of emphasis on the clinical side of medical schools.[76] The Association of American Medical Colleges in 2020 chose to remove the name "Abraham Flexner," whom they still regarded as the "father" of modern medical education, from its prestigious award for excellence because his racist opinions no longer reflected those of the Association.[77]

Final Assessment

Jim Crow, Progressive reforms, and a scientific revolution shaped the United States' modern health system. Jim Crow, as argued here, was the "root cause" for its distinctive development. Certainly, many factors contributed. Proof of the central role played by Jim Crow may never be convincing enough to some.

The case of the threatened takeover of Meharry Medical School by the Southern Governor's Conference beginning in 1948 offers an example of how convoluted Jim Crow health care politics could become and how difficult it can be to simply distinguish the heroes from the villains.[78] Meharry along with Howard were the only two Black medical schools to survive the Flexner era purge. In 1948 financial pressures threatened Meharry's closure. The Southern Governor's Conference approached the institution with a plan to buy it and assure its survival. Most southern states had already begun offering attractive scholarships to Meharry and Howard to Black medical school applicant residents. Meharry and Howard got the tuition dollars, and the student got his living and tuition costs covered. The Southern Governors, in turn, got to avoid the expected federal court decisions that would either force them to face the budget costs of building separate Black medical schools or the political cost of integrating their state-run ones. A Southern Regional Education Board was expected to negotiate the arrangements with Meharry's board. That produced an angry backlash among its alumni and Black medical leaders. The deal was never consummated.

In essence, during the Jim Crow era, there were no real winners. The efforts of the southern governors were briefly successful in delaying the opening of access of Black applicants to their state-operated schools. Soon afterward, all quietly submitted when faced with the threat of loss of the growing infusion of federal support for their medical schools. Federal efforts to expand health insurance coverage to assure something closer to universal access to care, however, met stiffer resistance. Health insurance in the United States remains still mired in the Jim Crow past.

CHAPTER THREE

The Death of Universal Health Care

JEAN COWSERT'S LIFETIME (1925–1967) included the creation of Social Security, the development of the private health insurance industry, and the implementation of Medicare. During that lifetime, other nations created arrangements to assure universal health care for their citizens. "Universal health care" (used interchangeably with the phrases "universal health coverage" and "universal health insurance") is defined as a system where all citizens can obtain health care without risking financial hardship from unaffordable out-of-pocket expenses.[1] Despite a century of attempts, the United States is the only affluent nation that has failed.

Jean's father, James Hugh Cowsert, played a bit part in that failure. He was an agent for the Life and Casualty Insurance Company of Tennessee. Founded in 1903, the company offered life insurance policies that predated those covering health care costs. At the time of Jean's birth, most paid out of pocket for their medical care. The indigent got what limited care they could from public and private charity clinics and hospitals. James sold two classes of life insurance reflecting what people could afford. "Industrial" life insurance policies, or "burial" insurance, provided small farmers and blue-collar workers with affordable premiums and a death benefit for their families to cover their funeral expenses. The "ordinary" policies catered to the middle class. In exchange for higher premiums, these policies provided a more generous benefit that could help defray the loss of the family's major breadwinner. Agents collected the premiums in person. That was the easy part. No one wanted to shame their families by having their body dumped in an unmarked pauper's grave. Agents were always on the road. Their livelihood depended on uncertain commissions. James died at fifty-two in 1939 when Jean was only fourteen. The Life and Casualty Company of Tennessee expanded during Jean's lifetime. Its new headquarters in Nashville, a thirty-one-story building completed in 1957, was the tallest in the Southeast.

Health insurance developed along two paths. It could be just a commercial product like life insurance where, given the benefits offered and risk, the insurance company determined an "actuarially fair" price. Those in poorer health would either face higher premiums or be judged uninsurable, just as with life insurance policies. Alternatively, health insurance could be a form of "social insurance," or collective concern for the less fortunate.[2] Governments or quasi-government agencies pursued this path, while companies like the Life and Casualty Company of Tennessee followed the commercial insurance one.

Industrial or "burial" life insurance policies became a growing business after the Civil War. For a small change premium, low-income workers could get policies that would pay a death benefit of one hundred dollars. Such policies were popular among low-income Black as well as white workers. Fraternal lodges offered similar benefits to members, but the industrial ones provided an aura of greater institutional reliability. Not anticipating Black demand and responding to Reconstruction Era antidiscrimination laws, white insurance companies sold the same policies to Black citizens as white. That ended in 1896, the same year as the *Plessy* Supreme Court decision.

Frederick L. Hoffman published his influential *Race Traits and Tendencies of the American Negro*.[3] That report, crammed with statistics and actuarial tables, provided "scientific racism" support for white supremacy and restricted Black access to life and health insurance coverage for half a century. According to Hoffman, Black people were racially inferior, perhaps doomed to extinction and uninsurable. Employed by Prudential Life Insurance, Hoffman's treatise helped insulate the company from antidiscrimination life insurance laws being passed in northern states. Prudential cut the death benefit on Black industrial policies by a third. Other life insurance companies either ceased writing policies for Black clients or offered them at higher premiums.[4] Universal health insurance implied that people from any racial group would be covered. Hoffman's report stiffened white resistance.

The commercial insurance path from life to health insurance, however, faced other barriers. An "insurable risk" was a rare, catastrophic, unpredictable, and easily identifiable event such as loss of life. Covering health care costs with commercial insurance was complicated. Health care costs depended on the decisions made by patients and providers. Insurance companies had no interest in exposing themselves to risks they knew little about and had no control over. Health insurance, was, after all, not really "insurance." It was an ugly duckling, a field dominated by social insurance schemes crafted by fraternal orders and community groups concerned with providing collective protection from the cost of illness and supporting the hospitals that provided such care.

As the cost of health care increased and arrangements for covering those costs grew, commercial insurance companies began to get interested. Large employers began to offer health benefits to their employees. Insurance companies responded by offering attractively priced health "insurance" products just to get their foot in the door—a "loss leader" that would enable them to sell the company's more conventional casualty and liability products.

For the commercial insurance companies focused on providing a benefit for a fair price, it was like a child being set loose in a candy store. Their major competitors were Blue Cross plans. These non-profit producer cooperative prepayment plans had been developed by hospitals. Envisioned as a voluntary form of social insurance, they offered employers a "community rate" for their employees. In calculating that rate, the Blue Cross plan just divided their total payments to hospitals for care of their enrollees by the total number of enrollees. Such a rate spread the costs evenly across everyone, as envisioned by a social insurance program. Dock workers that lived rough lives resulting in high medical costs paid the same premium as school-teachers. True to form, the commercial insurance companies lured lower cost employer groups such as schoolteachers away with lower premiums. Faced with the threat of bankruptcy from being left with only the costliest employer groups, the Blue Cross plans switched paths. They abandoned community rating. Blue Cross plans began to set rates based on the cost experience of each employer group, just as the commercial insurance companies did. Those most in need of such coverage would be those least able to afford it. Voluntary insurance ceased to be a realistic way to achieve universal care.

The vision of health insurance in the United States as a form of social insurance faded and the focus of both voluntary and commercial forms of health insurance shifted to just capturing profitable business opportunities. That involved finding ways to shift the adverse risks onto one's competitors. It could be done through selective marketing, benefit design, cost sharing, and selective provider contracting. (Some examples come from national health insurance proposals, described later in this chapter.) Supported by labor unions and management, the private pay employer-based health insurance market boomed after World War II. It expanded further after 1965, absorbing an increasing share of the publicly financed health insurance business created by the Medicare and Medicaid programs for the elderly and the indigent.[5]

The vision of universal care died a slow death. Racial ideology played a central role in that death. It shaped the segregated division of insurance. It took for granted the Confederate post-Reconstruction "lost cause" myths that served as justification for its Jim Crow structure. The ideology was skillfully invoked by the vested interests created in that structure to defeat a century of initiatives attempting to create universal care.

Jim Crow Health Insurance

Health insurance, just as schooling, housing, criminal justice, and the delivery of health care, adapted to the structure of Jim Crow. The same nested cages described earlier in Figure 1 (page 4) constrained national health insurance policy, local community insurance options, and the choices individuals had about where to get care. It divided the third-party payment of care between a private insurance system and a publicly financed one. The private insurance system served mostly white populations and the more affluent. The publicly financed system served the indigent and a disproportionate share of the Black population. Since Jean Cowsert's birth in 1925, that basic divide has never changed. Those providing care to predominantly Black and low-income populations are paid less for their services and their patients have more restricted choices about where to get care. Health insurance reforms have done little to change this. Some have exacerbated the disparities in care since efforts to control costs and improve efficiencies have focused on the publicly financed arrangements for the low-income population, leaving the arrangements provided for the more affluent and predominantly white population untouched.

The best way to eliminate the disparate impact of a two-class system of care is to eliminate it. Other wealthier democracies have adopted this approach—a single universal health system. The cost is spread evenly. Everyone is covered. You do not face the problem of denying care to those that are not covered or spreading the cost of that care across those that are covered. The costs for everyone are covered by taxation, employer, and beneficiary contributions, or some combination of these. If everyone participates in the same plan the adverse risk selection and the inadequate coverage problems disappear. This obvious solution has been adopted by all affluent democracies except the United States. Only the Republic of South Africa shares a similar patchwork insurance arrangement. Both countries share a history of racial division—Jim Crow in the United States and Apartheid in South Africa. Both countries pay a similar price for that history—a fragmented nonuniversal system of insurance that costs more and is less effective.

International comparisons long documented the price the United States pays for its fragmented insurance system. A recent report by the Commonwealth Fund compares the United States to ten other high income countries that chose the path to universal care.[6] On measures of access, administrative efficiency, equity and health care outcomes, the United States ranks well below these other countries. The United States excels only in measures of the "process of care," or how complete the care provided is, *once one gained access to a provider*. On this indicator, the United States ranks second among these eleven countries. In other words, it is the financing system surrounding that care that results in its overall poor marks. The United States spends more for care but gets less in return. Despite a century of attempts, the United States failed to follow the path to universal care, and race played a role.

Redemption of the Lost Cause

Most explanations of this failure to achieve universal care in the United States focus on: (1) the nation's peculiar ideological culture, (2) the powerful influence of interest groups (e.g., the American Medical

Association (AMA) and, more recently, the private insurance industry), and (3) a political system where broader public interests are more fragmented, making only minor incremental change possible.[7] The few that mention race do not dig back far enough.[8] In essence, the Confederate "lost cause myth" cast a shadow over the nation's debate over universal care. The nineteenth-century version of that myth recast the Civil War as a struggle to preserve state rights and a moral order, not as a battle over slavery. It provided the justification for the perpetuation of white supremacy and the imposition of Jim Crow. It persists as a powerful force in national politics.[9] Its nineteenth century roots are visible in the history of Mobile, Alabama. The lost cause myths, well concealed, shaped the subsequent century long debate over universal health insurance. Those myths just became part of the conventional wisdom about the "American way." That way valued private control and labeled public control as "socialism." As publicly financed services shifted to private hands, the problems posed by racial segregation and inequities got buried.

The struggle over health insurance transformed the lost cause myths into campaign slogans. They became the sound bites used to defeat efforts to expand health insurance in the United States. What made them so powerful was that the link with the Confederate past was so well concealed. Ingrained into popular wisdom, Jim Crow arguments savaged five separate health insurance reform initiatives over the last century.

"We Take Care of Our Own"

Social solidarity extends only to "your own." It began with mutual protection associations established by immigrant groups, Black communities, churches, guilds, and labor unions in the nineteenth century. The "lost cause" myths of the Confederacy strengthened that idea among Southern whites. It surfaced in the implementation of Medicare in 1966. A universal health insurance program for seniors, its implementation became the first test of the Civil Rights Act of 1964 prohibition against the use of federal funds in any organization that discriminated based on race.

A small hospital in Texas became a focus of concern of civil rights activists and a source of embarrassment to President Johnson. While it claimed it did not discriminate, its patient census was all white in a service area that included a large Black population. Leon Bernstein, an experienced hospital administrator hired to assist HEW in the implementation of the Medicare program, was sent by Assistant Secretary Wilbur Cohen to address this aberration. The hospital's administrator met his questioning about the hospital's failure to serve Black patients with indignation: "Why, they take care of their own!"[10] Indeed, many members of local Black communities would not have disagreed. In self-defense a large network of Black hospitals had developed in both the North and South. Despite limited resources they were revered by most community members as "their own." The closure of almost all of them following desegregation after the passage of the Medicare Act, was an ambivalent experience in all of their communities.[11] It was a well ingrained view dating back to the lodges and fraternal orders that had set prepayment arrangements for their members. These groups resisted early state efforts to set up government sponsored health insurance for blue collar industrial workers.[12] Labor unions similarly resisted. Just as with the lodges, unions bargained benefits that became too attractive a recruiting tool to give up.

"The Voluntary Way Is the American Way"

"Voluntarism" is the notion that social welfare needs could best be addressed by organizations independent of the state and supported by private voluntary charitable contributions. Such a model of ownership of hospitals flourished in the Jim Crow era. The early forms of health insurance or "prepayment" followed the same ownership model. Mutual protection organizations such as private lodges and fraternal groups, first began such prepayment plans for their members. Later the voluntary hospitals themselves formed similar arrangements. These would evolve into the Blue Cross and Blue Shield network of plans that still account for a large share of the private health insurance market. While such ownership patterns are taken for granted in the United States, they are viewed as a puzzling anachronism in most other affluent nations. Such ownership shifted public control to the private control of white elites. Even elections to public office in most of the former Confederacy were controlled by a white-only voluntary membership association—the state Democratic Party. In Alabama, for example, the Democratic Party functioned like a private club that excluded Black members. Only party members could vote in the primary elections. Given the Democratic party's dominance, in Alabama and other states in the South, whoever won the primary won the general election. Thurgood Marshall and the NAACP challenged this obvious Black disenfranchisement. That led to the US Supreme Court rejecting the constitutionality of such private primaries 1944 (*Smith v. Allwright,* US 321 649 [1944]). Marshall viewed it as his most important civil rights legal victory. Similar "disenfranchisement" was taken for granted in the voluntary hospital sector. It determined not just who served on its board but who had privileges on its medical staff. Voluntary hospitals excluded not just Black patients but those not of the same ethnic or religious background. Catholic hospitals were established not just to serve as a place for Catholic patients but to employ either Irish Catholic or Italian Catholic physicians. Similarly, Jewish hospitals were created to serve the Russian or German Jewish physicians. Such ethnic and religious exclusions did not begin to break down until after Medicare's implementation blocked the exclusion of Black physicians from medical privileges.

The voluntary model, exclusively serving members of a particular racial or ethnic group, shaped the development of health insurance or prepayment. Fraternal orders, religious congregations and immigrant groups all looked after their members and served as private welfare systems. Freed enslaved persons and their descendants formed similar voluntary mutual self-protection associations. The community health center movement as noted by one of its leaders built on these past efforts: "In Mound Bayou, Mississippi, the Knights and Daughters of Tabor pooled their resources and built a forty-bed modern hospital in 1941 in one of the poorest counties in the nation. It was without a doubt the best hospital for Blacks in Mississippi at that time. . . . In my own family we belonged to a similar order that looked after families facing crises. My grandfather and great grandfather were active members in such organizations, My father who was doing well contributed two pigs a year to the community larder each year. The community owned these resources which would keep a couple of families out of trouble for a year. Almost everybody in the 1930s and 1940s were members."[13]Just as the Knights and Daughters of Tabor did, all the groups looked after their own and began negotiating with physicians for annual payment for the care they provided their members. Hospitals borrowed the idea to create a similar voluntary community arranged to help cover participants hospital costs. In other nations this evolved into a government insurance program. In contrast, in the United States the existence of such voluntary arrangements was used to argue against the need for a government program. Government control was defined as "socialism."

The AMA launched a well-orchestrated and financed campaign to attack Truman's National Health Insurance plan that would be financed through Social Security. They attacked the Truman Administration as "followers of the Moscow party line" and labeled their health insurance plan "Un-American."[14] The "voluntary way is the American way" the AMA argued. More than a million pamphlets and billboards promoted the message: "Compulsory health insurance: political medicine is bad medicine for America" in one of the most well-funded political action campaigns in history.[15] Included in the promotional campaign was a reproduction of British artist Luke Fildes's painting *The Doctor*. It portrays a doctor (white) caring for a sick child (white) in his home late at night with the warning "keep politics out of this picture."[16] Only Black doctors, excluded from hospital privileges and forced to care for their patients in their homes rather than in increasingly well-equipped modern hospitals, could appreciate the irony of such posters. Truman's proposal never had a chance.

"Freedom of Choice"

The Confederate lost cause myth portrayed individual freedom as America's most precious value. The myth portrayed the federal government as the evil destroyer of that freedom. After all, why shouldn't an individual be free to choose health insurance the way one chooses beer, cigarettes, or cereal? Isn't that what capitalism is all about? The problem is that health insurance is not just another product in a free market; it serves, no matter what the ownership patterns, as a form of mutual protection or social insurance. Treating insurance as just another product in the free market (1) undermines its usefulness, (2) makes achieving universal care impossible, and (3) exacerbates the racial segregation and disparities in care.

For example, the more health insurance caters to the specific needs of an individual, the less it spreads the risks. If you are young and healthy and cannot avoid paying for health insurance, you want an inexpensive plan that perhaps just covers catastrophic costs. If you are planning to have a baby, you will want full coverage of maternity and pediatric services. If you are suffering from the early stages of Alzheimer's, you will want good long-term care benefits. As the health insurance market gets divided up this way, the premiums an individual pays begin to reflect the costs they incur. Such plans stop being insurance that pools the risks to assure that everyone will be taken care of and just becomes a payment plan like a loan for a car or a mortgage for a house. Unlike the decision to purchase a car or a house, however, the cost of one's medical care tends to be inversely related to an individual's ability to pay for it. The premiums for those with high costs will become just as unaffordable as the out-of-pocket expenses they will incur *without* insurance. The idea of social insurance was that everyone would share the costs for the sickest and most vulnerable. That was the idea of "universal social insurance" and the "community rating" idea as it was used by the early Blue Cross plans. Freedom of choice killed both and left a nation with almost as great racial health disparities today as in its Jim Crow past.

Medicare was the exception. During the effort to desegregate hospitals with the implementation of Medicare, freedom of choice became the rallying cry of those that wanted to preserve segregation in hospitals. By the time of Medicare's implementation in 1966, most public and medical school owned hospitals had been desegregated.[17] Only the voluntary ones, the bulk of hospital facilities in the United States who were less dependent on federal funding and whose nondiscrimination requirements were more ambiguous lagged. Even after Medicare forced the removal of racially restrictive signs, the racial segregation of many services and facilities remained unchanged. Fearing retaliation, few Black patients or doctors dared break the now invisible color barriers. Hospital leaders of previously segregated facilities did not see any problem with this. Individuals should be "free to choose." That "choice" should be left up to the patient in consultation with their physician. The hospital had no business in interfering in that sacred private relationship between the doctor and their patient. They should have freedom of choice and not be forced into racially integrated floors and services. This was the final battle that Dr. Cowsert found herself engaged in. It was also the rallying cry in the battle against "compulsory" (universal) health insurance that still rages.

"Cost Control and the Privatization of Insurance"

Health insurance in the United States developed along the commercial rather than social insurance path. The only breach came with the implementation of the Medicare legislation in 1966. It had the potential of ending the Jim Crow health care and expanding into a universal insurance program. A lost cause backlash, however, crushed that promise. That backlash focused on the seemingly racially neutral initiatives of: (1) redesigning payments to give providers an incentive to control costs and (2) privatizing health insurance. As will be described in the next section, the same lost cause strategies that helped put an end to Reconstruction helped put an end to universal care. Universal care in the United States became the ultimate "cold case."

The Elusive Pursuit of Universal Care

If you want to tell the story of "structural racism" in health care, you have to "follow the money." Health insurance is about the flow of that money. The details about each of these five offensives to achieve universal care have been fleshed out in other books.[18] A more detailed summary of this account is provided elsewhere.[19] Table 1 outlines the five major offensives. What is remarkable is how much of the lost cause myths got translated into strategies to defeat all of them.

The Death of Progressive Era Efforts (1896–1934)

In the shadow of *Plessy*, two groups shaped the health insurance debate: those just concerned with "taking care of their own," and an interest group of Progressive Era professionals and politicians concerned about broader reforms. Lodges and fraternal orders, sharing common racial and ethnic identities tried to serve their members by contracting with physicians. As the scale of manufacturing grew, Progressive era political and professional leaders tried to design health care insurance solutions for industrial settings.

TABLE 1. HOW JIM CROW STALLED UNIVERSAL HEALTH CARE INITIATIVES, 1896 TO 2022

	1896–1934	1934–1954	1954–1973	1973–1994	1994–2022
Strategies for preserving Jim Crow and blocking universal health care (UHC)	"We take care of our own." Consumer adaptation to Jim Crow.	"The voluntary way is the American way." Provider adaptation to Jim Crow.	People should be "free to choose." No GOVERNMENT-IMPOSED INTEGRATION.	"Management is the solution." Segregation in the guise of cost control (e.g., HMOs and DRGs).	"Government is the problem." Free market circumvention of integration and civil rights law.
Key special interest opponents of UHC	Lodges and trade unions	AHA and AMA	AMA and Southern segregationists	Private insurance coalitions	Emerging private sector insurers, suppliers, and providers.
UHC proposals and their outcomes	Model state legislation supporting shared financing by worker, employer, and state of industrial workers. (American Association of Labor Legislation) **FAILED**	National Universal Health Insurance funded by Social Security. (Roosevelt and Truman) **FAILED**	Medicare Social Security Act of 1965, coverage for those over 65. (Johnson) **PASSED BUT EXPANSION TO THE REST OF THE POPULATION STALLED**	The Health Security Bill, expanded coverage through managed care networks. (Clinton) **FAILED**	Affordable Care Act of 2010, expanded Medicaid and private coverage, individually mandated coverage, and preexisting condition protection. (Obama) **PASSED BUT FUTURE UNCERTAIN**

From David Barton Smith, "The Pandemic Challenge: End Separate and Unequal Health Care," *American Journal of the Medical Sciences* 360, no. 1: 109–11. Reprinted with permission from the Southern Society for Clinical Investigation, 2020.

Theodore Roosevelt, as the presidential candidate of the newly formed Progressive "Bull Moose" Party in 1912, was the first to nationally promote the idea of health insurance. Although never fleshed out, it was an approach like the legislative plan advocated by the American Association of Labor Legislation (AALL), a Progressive social reform group. In a disastrous miscalculation, Roosevelt attempted to capture the votes of white Southerners by refusing to seat Black delegates at the party's convention. Black leaders were enraged. As President, Theodore Roosevelt had previously accepted the disenfranchisement of Black people in the South. Overall, his actions and words suggest he had absorbed most of the vision of the white supremacy lost cause mythology.[20]

The American Association of Labor Legislation (AALL) during World War I sponsored state legislation to provide health care to industrial workers supported by matching funds from the state, the employers, and the employees. Lodges had already begun providing such protection for their members and objected. They contracted with physicians to provide care for their members for a fixed amount per year. Despite the opposition of local medical societies, this approach to assuring access to care grew rapidly and many assumed it was the way most care would be financed in the future. They saw no reason to undermine their influence in recruiting new members by substituting "compulsory governmental paternalism for private voluntary fraternalism." National leaders of the AMA were generally supportive of the AALL proposals.[21] It would be the last time the AMA would support such legislation. State and local medical societies, however, worked effectively with the lodges to block state legislation.

In the end, both victors in this battle had fatal flaws. For lodge medicine those flaws involved adverse risk selection and limited contracting leverage. Lodges providing health care benefits attracted and kept members that needed care. That raised the cost of membership or made it more difficult to find physicians that would contract with the lodge to provide care to their members. The lodges also faced hostile medical societies and hospital associations that functioned as quasi monopolies. The local medical societies defined physicians engaged in lodge practices as unethical. As a result, the local medical society rejected them from membership and the hospitals refused to grant them privileges.

For the voluntary producer cooperative approach to health insurance promoted by the medical societies and hospitals, the fatal flaw came from just the reverse—*their power to avoid adverse risk selection.* This came to a head in a final Progressive effort to find a solution to the problem. The Committee on the Cost of Medical Care (CCMC), established in 1927, was a five-year effort to figure out how the growing cost of medical care could best be financed to meet the needs of the American people. Supported by eight private foundations, including the Rosenwald Fund, it was aided by all the major white professional associations (American Medical Association, American Dental Association, American Hospital Association, etc.), the US Public Health Service, and state and local health departments. The "Committee" itself consisted of fifty leaders including private medical practitioners, dentists, representatives of institutional providers, public health, and a few other public sector representatives. All were white and none were politicians. There was nothing in its composition that would raise objections among lost cause ideologues. The effort produced twenty-seven professionally researched reports. Detailed information was collected on the problems of white access to care, the ability to pay for it, and how best to address these problems. Black participants were excluded from the major survey because the staff of the CCMC concluded that "the procedure adopted could not procure satisfactory information from Negro families."[22] As far as these reports were concerned, the need for Black care did not exist.

The Committee's final majority recommendations proposed creating a more organized group practice form of delivery and placing financing on a group payment basis through private insurance or taxation. These tentative, incremental steps were hardly earth shattering. Yet, medical practice representatives on the Committee objected to any suggestion that pay should shift from fee for service to some kind of "contract payment." *JAMA* in its editorial on the report blasted the majority recommendations as "representing the forces of great foundations, public health officialdom and social theory—even socialism and communism—inciting revolution."[23] Even the *New York Times*, a presumably more objective source, heralded the release of the report in its headline "Socialized Medicine Is Urged in Survey."[24]

The final report left unresolved whether to pursue a voluntary insurance approach or a government taxation approach to financing. That issue bitterly divided members of the Committee and its staff. Indeed, the Committee unanimously agreed on only one issue: *commercial insurance companies should never be allowed to play a role in the financing of health care*. All members recognized that, with their entry, neither the voluntary nor the taxation social insurance approach could survive. The battle between government and voluntary financing of health insurance would play out over the next twenty years. The commercial insurance sector's role in financing health care would come later.

The Demise of Social Security–Based National Health Insurance (1934–1954)

Inaugurated President in March 1933. Franklin Roosevelt needed immediate action in the face of the crisis posed by the Great Depression. A workgroup quickly drafted a social security bill. They debated inclusion of health insurance. Aware of the hostile reception the CCMC majority recommendations had received, they concluded that health insurance was a "very complex and controversial subject that might jeopardize speed and favorable congressional action on the committee's recommendations."[25] Roosevelt concurred.

With the help of former CCMC staff advocating for the voluntary insurance approach, hospitals and medical societies filled the void, creating what became the Blue Cross and Blue Shield system. Borrowing from some of the ideas of the lodge medicine movement, they created a network of hospital and medical producer cooperative insurance plans. It rapidly expanded employer-based insurance coverage. This disproportionately benefited the white population but relegated many Black families to the public indigent care system. Former CCMC staff supportive of the taxation approach to health insurance worked within the newly established social security system to promote such proposals. President Truman would introduce a revised bill calling for the creation of a compulsory national health insurance system funded by payroll taxes in 1945. He argued that the only change in the organization of care would be that the care received would no longer depend on how much you could afford to pay at the time. The American people, Truman argued "will not be frightened off from health insurance because some people have misnamed it 'socialized medicine.'"[26] As noted earlier, however, the AMA lobbying effort succeeded in doing just that.

Civil Rights Revival of Federal Financing and the Creation of Medicare (1954–1973)

The *Brown* decision, the Civil Rights Act of 1964, and the political pressures of civil rights activists transformed what was possible. At the high-water mark of the civil rights movement, these forces propelled the passage of Medicare in 1965 and shaped its implementation. The only physicians to attend the signing ceremony with President Johnson at Truman's Presidential Library were members of the National Medical Association, the African American medical association, which had worked to support its passage. Representatives of the hospital and health insurance industry were notably absent.

Medicare's impact was profound. Using Title VI, the untested provision of the Civil Rights Act of 1964 that prohibited the allocation of federal funds to any institution or program that discriminated based on race segregated patterns persistent for a century in voluntary hospitals were eliminated in three months.[27] Most gross racial disparities in use of hospital and physician services disappeared within a few years.[28] Racial and economic disparities in basic measures of health narrowed in the first fifteen years after Medicare's passage.[29]

The assumption of most involved in Medicare's implementation was that the program for the elderly was just the "foot in the door" and that it would lead quickly to an expansion of coverage under Social Security.[30] A last-minute inclusion of a state-administered program for the indigent, Medicaid was assumed by most liberals to be temporary and soon discarded. These state indigent-care programs had always been a shabby excuse for mainstream care. Liberal conventional wisdom dismissed them as "poor care for poor people" that would soon be replaced with Medicare expansions. It did not happen. The last extension of the Medicare Act came with the 1972 amendment during the Nixon Administration to cover those under sixty-five who were permanently disabled or suffering from end-stage renal disease. In the growing conservative backlash against civil rights reforms, Medicaid became the major vehicle for expanding coverage, blocking any realistic reduction in the racial and economic segregation and disparities in care. Medicare and Medicaid also became targets for the redesign of reimbursement to control cost that also increased segregation and disparities.

Redesigning Payment to Control Costs (1973–1994)

In the backlash to the civil rights era efforts, the policy focus shifted to controlling costs. For Medicare, the focus shifted to designing a system of fixed payment to hospitals per discharge by "diagnostically related groups" or DRGs. The basic idea of DRGs was to provide a hospital with a financial incentive to limit costly inpatient hospital use. For Medicaid the focus shifted to designing a system of payment to physicians for care by capitated rates. The basic idea of capitated rates for physicians was to give them a financial incentive to limit the services they provided patients. While their success in stemming overall cost increases in these two programs is debatable, the two payment systems did succeed in partially re-segregating and adding to disparities in the care provided.

Diagnostically Related Groups (DRGs)

DRGs provided hospitals with a financial incentive to shift much of the care that had been provided in acute hospitals back into home and outpatient settings. Hospital costs account for the largest proportion of total health care expenditures. The easiest way to reduce costs, one could argue, would be to reduce hospital use. Giving hospitals a financial incentive to reduce admissions and lengths of stay would seem an easy way for payers to reduce costs. A DRG payment system gives a hospital a payment that would on the average cover the reasonable cost of care for such a case. If a hospital can reduce the length of stay or treat the patient on an outpatient basis, it makes more money. It leaves the insurance provider with "clean hands," shifting responsibility for sometimes risky cost saving decisions onto the hospital providers.

It is not clear whether this in the end saved money. Some of the cost got shifted to outpatient settings and long-term care facilities. Premature discharges, encouraged by these incentives, resulted in readmissions that added to hospital costs.[31] The bottom line is that while DRG payments reduced lengths of stay and overall hospital days per 1,000 population, it also increased acuity, which added to costs. Even though the volume of hospital inpatient care dropped, total inpatient hospital costs per person in the United States are still the highest in the world.[32]

What DRGs did do was partially resegregate care. The reduced occupancy in hospitals enabled many, including those in Mobile, Alabama, to convert to all private rooms. This ended the requirement for racially blind assignment to double occupancy rooms that had been the decisive test of Title VI compliance. The shortened length of stays also shifted much of the care onto outpatient and long-term care providers. In low income and mostly Black communities these resources were in short supply and of lower quality than in more affluent white neighborhoods.[33] Hospital segregation is lower than residential segregation, but nursing home segregation is higher than both.[34] Shifting the amount of care from less segregated settings (hospitals) to more segregated ones (nursing homes and residences) increased the overall degree of segregation of care. In other words, care became more separate and unequal. The acuity of those left in hospital beds also increased. DRGs reduced the use of inpatient hospital care, the health care resource most effectively desegregated and relegated it to those, least likely to be socially aware of their integrated surroundings.

Capitation

In introducing the Health Maintenance Organization Act of 1973, Richard Nixon argued that: "under traditional systems doctors and hospitals are paid in effect on a piecework basis. The more illnesses they treat—and the more services they render—the more they make . . . There is no economic incentive to concentrate on keeping them healthy."[35] The Clinton administration, two decades later, would borrow Nixon's argument in constructing their Health Security Plan of 1993. The impact of HMOs and capitated forms of payment were not as simple or as upbeat as Nixon's statement or what the proponents of the Clinton plan suggested. What is remarkable is how the idea that HMOs were doing something special to "maintain" health and reduce health care costs continued long after the evidence no longer made the argument plausible.

What should have been more troubling was the hold this form of payment would grow to have over state Medicaid programs.

Pennsylvania, an early adopter, for example, created a program with an Orwellian name, "Health Choices." Recipients did not really have choices; they could pick between a few Medicaid only mostly for-profit HMOs that limited the choice of physicians and hospitals recipients could use. These HMOs were paid a risk-adjusted capitated rate for the care they provided, and that rate was determined by assuring that the overall cost of the program or the overall "community capitation" would be fixed. Similar models were adopted for Medicaid programs in most states but never quite caught on in the Medicare program that still offered the choice of a traditional option. The Clinton Health Security Bill of 1994, relying heavily on HMO contracting in the face of rising opposition to such arrangements from those with private insurance never had a chance.

Privatizing Public Payment Programs (1994–present)

The next predictable move in the chess game by the lost cause ideologues was to shoot for full privatization. As Reagan argued in his first inauguration as president, "Government isn't the solution; it is the problem."[36] In the resulting political environment, liberal concern with expanding health care coverage could be achieved only in exchange for expanding privatization. Expanding Medicare benefits with HMO options, insurance coverage for children, drug benefits for seniors, and, ultimately, the Obama plan for expanding coverage to the uninsured, were all bought at the price of an expanded role for the commercial insurance sector.

Part of the price in an expanded role for the private insurance sector are increased segregation and disparities in care. Title VI prohibited the use of federal funds in institutions and programs that discriminate based on race. This was easy to enforce in the implementation of Medicare since there was only one program and no choice. However, as health insurance programs becomes privatized, discriminatory intent in the segregation and disparities that result become invisible. If, for example, low-income minorities flock to a Medicare private option that eliminates co-pays in exchange for a restricted list of providers, it will result in a higher degree of segregation and probably increased disparities in the care. It would be hard to argue, however, that it is a violation of any of the antidiscrimination provisions of civil rights law. There are no "white only" signs, no explicit racist policies, not even any "smoking gun" racist comments by gatekeepers. Individuals were "free to choose" the option that best fitted their needs. Should those designing this insurance option targeting this specific market segment, e.g., low-income minorities, receive criticism or approval? Only an insurance program that eliminated all economic barriers would eliminate the potential for economic segregation and disparities.

The more serious problems that privatization soon created in assuring expanded coverage were a lack of affordable insurance and rising un-insurance rates. This raised questions about its long-term viability. In 1989 the Heritage Foundation, a conservative think tank with an ideological stake in preserving a privatized solution to universal coverage, outlined a plan to address these problems.[37] It included three key elements: (1) a community rating plan requiring insurers to make plans affordable regardless of health status (e.g., no exclusion of preexisting conditions), (2) an individual mandate requiring everyone, healthy or not, have coverage, and (3) subsidies to low-income individuals so everyone could afford coverage. A group of health economists weighed in arguing that such a plan was the only avenue for "responsible national health insurance."[38] The only alternatives were either (1) reliance on an employer mandate that faced growing employer resistance and would leave many uncovered or (2) a "Medicare for all" approach that would face fierce conservative opposition. The basic outline of the Heritage Foundation proposals became Governor Romney's health insurance bill for Massachusetts passed in 2006.[39] Nuances aside, this is what became the national

Patient Protection and Affordable Care Act passed in December 2009. The major difference was that it was proposed by America's first Black president who was a Democrat. Labeled disparagingly by Republicans as "Obama Care," not a single Republican voted for it and the party did everything they could to block its implementation. After a decade of heated opposition, never producing an alternative to what was originally their own creation, it has ceased to be a target of Republican attacks. Following the lead of conservative think tanks, it helped expand coverage by further privatizing it. It did nothing to alter the existing fragmented insurance system. Its future in contributing to or alleviating segregation and disparities in care remains to be written.

Conclusion

There is always room for optimism. We are, in the face of a seemingly never-ending COVID pandemic, all in it together. The health of any individual depends on the heath of everyone. That is the basic argument for social insurance as opposed to a commercial insurance free market approach. Perhaps this can lead organized medicine, a century long laggard in promoting universal care, to finally question the hollow rhetoric that has supported the status quo of Jim Crow health care. Something as simple as just a uniform payment structure would not just cut costs but help end the tiered segregated system of care that persists.

Some, echoing the lost cause position, argue that the failure to achieve universal health care is fine since such care is an infringement on individual freedom.[40] Most Americans, however, believe that people who need care should get it and reject such a conclusion. A poll of registered voters in the United State in 2020 indicated that 69 percent supported providing Medicare to every American, including 46 percent of Republicans.[41] The results of this survey are consistent with earlier ones. Despite such support, few policy makers give such an option much of a chance. A patchwork of incremental extensions in coverage has taken place while preserving a segregated and unequal system of care. While the health care Jim Crow labels have disappeared, its financial structure remains in Mobile, Alabama as well as the rest of the nation.

PART II

Mobile

CHAPTER FOUR

The Lost Cause

JEAN COWSERT SET UP HER PRACTICE in Mobile at a time that racial relations were not that different than those of Mobile's diverse antebellum past. A microcosm of the American experience, Mobile would cycle through many rising dreams of a multiracial democracy only to be crushed. It was a colonial outpost fought over by France, Spain, and England. Indigenous Americans, decimated by the infectious diseases that European colonist brought with them, were forced off their land. That land was made available for exploitation by a few white settlers who accumulated great wealth from cotton. Mobile, at the center of this "cotton kingdom," exported the crop and imported the enslaved persons essential for its production. The city mixed the ambience of the wild west with all the excesses of early capitalism. It never fully recovered from the destruction of the Confederacy during the Civil War. The lost cause narrative would in the end dominate, placing blame on the victims of slavery and those that tried to assure their full citizenship. Jim Crow's grip on Mobile would become absolute by the beginning of the twentieth century.

Mobile before the Civil War

Mobile Bay, thirty-five miles long and eight to twenty miles wide, is the terminus of the second largest river basin system in North America. That basin includes the Tombigbee, Black Warrior, Alabama, Mobile, Coosa, Tallapoosa, and Cahaba rivers, which drain more than two thirds of the land mass of Alabama.[1] Four of Alabama's largest cities—Birmingham, Tuscaloosa, Montgomery, and Mobile—as well as a large portion of the Atlanta metropolitan area rely upon it for drinking and wastewater assimilation. Its diverse ecosystem, once described as "America's Amazon," is now threatened just as is Brazil's.

The Bay lured settlement by indigenous peoples thousands of years before European explorers.[2] Hunter-gatherers attracted by the Bay's shellfish evolved into permanent trading and agricultural centers. Abandoned ceremonial mounds now dot a region extending from the Gulf Coast to as far north as Iowa and Ohio. Its first French explorer mistakenly named the island at the entrance to Mobile Bay "Massacre Island." Storm erosion had exposed a pile of human skeletons from a ceremonial burial mound misinterpreted as the site of a massacre.[3] It was later renamed "Dauphin Island," the title of the eldest son of the king of France, in the hope of attracting French settlers.

The French, jockeying for control of the region with Spain and England, set up Mobile as the capital of French Louisiana in 1702. Disease ridden, it had trouble attracting settlers and remained little more than a trading post. The English bought the area through the Treaty of Paris in 1763. Spain captured Mobile in 1780, and then returned it to France as part of the Louisiana territory in 1802. A year later that territory was then sold to the United States and all disputes over its ownership settled in the 1819 Florida Treaty with Spain. The city, with its French, Spanish, Creole (mixed European and Black Caribbean), free Black, and enslaved residents remained culturally diverse and distinct from the rest of Alabama.

Infectious diseases (smallpox, bubonic plague, chickenpox, cholera, typhus, tuberculosis) went with the Europeans to the Americas and devastated the largely unexposed indigenous population.
These diseases led to 55 million deaths, killing off almost 90 percent
of indigenous populations between 1500 and 1700.[4] The loss of population was so high, it contributed to the myth of America as a "vir-
gin wilderness." Settlements vanished, forests recovered, and long
abandoned fields left the illusion of an untouched beauty open for
exploitation. That pandemic loss lingers on. The per capita COV-
ID-19 death toll of the Navajo Nation is higher than that of any state.[5]
"Deaths of despair" among the Native American population (suicide,
drug overdoses, alcoholism) exceed the rates of any other racial or
ethnic group in the United States.

This decimation helped European appropriation of native lands
and the importation of enslaved labor to profitably exploit it. Africans shared much of the European partial immunity to the same infectious diseases. The transatlantic slave trade shipped about twelve
million enslaved persons between the sixteenth and nineteenth centuries with about 1.5 million dying in transit.[6]

The transatlantic slave trade also supplied some ironic revenge
that could only be fully appreciated by Africans surviving the Middle Passage and indigenous Americans subjected to the forced removal from their lands in Alabama. It brought yellow fever to the
Caribbean.[7] Europeans did not share the partial immunity that their
African enslaved cargo did. In 1803, Napoleon sent 40,000 troops
to Hispaniola to crush the Haitian slave rebellion. Yellow fever decimated the French expedition and only one-third survived to retreat.

That same year, unwilling to cling to what seemed a worthless, fatally disease-ridden region and in need of funds, Napoleon sold the
Louisiana territory to the United States. The purchase extended the
United States from the Gulf to the Canadian border. It helped insulate Westward development from conflicts with stronger European

powers. The purchase also increased the demand for enslaved persons to work the newly gotten fertile indigenous American lands in what would become Mississippi and Alabama.

Mobile stayed the center of the slave trade in Alabama until the 1850s. Slavery played a central role in the nation's economy, not just in the few cotton-growing states such as Alabama. Cotton represented the nation's largest export and the capital invested in enslavement to produce it exceeded that of all the railroads and factories in the nation.[8] Slavery reached into every aspect of the nation's economic development and the logic of its "free" enterprise system. Enslaved people as property were used as collateral for bank loans to buy more land and more humans in a highly leveraged business dependent on bank financing. Success depended on large scale efficient cotton production. The amount of cotton picked per day per enslaved person, according to one account, increased by 400 percent between 1810s and 1850s because of the "disciplinary technologies brought to bear by plantation management."[9] In other words, torture usually inflicted with a whip. Many of the nation's top universities—Brown, Columbia, Dartmouth, Harvard, Pennsylvania, Princeton, and Yale among others—partially owed their existence to the endowments from family fortunes made in the transatlantic slave trade and cotton.[10] That close financial connection to slavery had the predictable effect of shaping a hostile view of abolitionists at Northern universities.

Georgetown University, for example, faced serious pre–Civil War financial difficulties. This led to the sale of 272 enslaved people owned by two school presidents, who were Jesuit priests, to help pay off its debts.[11] The enslaved persons were shipped to New Orleans, families broken up and many sold to plantations with reputations for brutality. All regions, including elite northern universities, were well embedded in the national slave-cotton economy.

An Act of Congress abolished the transatlantic slave trade in 1807. Slavers began to rely on domestic production and relocation of enslaved people within the United States. Troubled by the successful slave rebellion in Haiti, buyers preferred the safer "domesticated" product. This increased the value of enslaved females of child-bearing age. Slave owners along the eastern seaboard where profits from ownership were declining raised no objection to the Act. They could cash in their investment profitably, just as Georgetown University had. Domestic slavers shipped about one million enslaved persons in the first half of the nineteenth century from the East Coast to the new cotton-growing areas of the Deep South.

Slavers shipped many captured people by sea from Maryland, Virginia, and the Carolinas to Mobile for sale. Mobile's slave market for most of the antebellum period was on the west side of Royal Street between St. Louis and St. Anthony.[12] An adjacent three-story prison barrack housed enslaved persons between auctions. The conditions were atrocious and bothered even community members untroubled by the institution of slavery. These holding pens were removed and placed on the city's periphery to make them less publicly conspicuous.

Mobile, still a rebellious frontier seaport, did not always follow the federal law prohibiting transatlantic slave trade. For some, it offered an irresistible opportunity for handsome profits while thumbing their nose at federal officials. Timothy Meaher and his two brothers, who had moved from Maine and owned sawmills, plantations, and enslaved persons, jumped at such an opportunity after a wager. They recruited William Sanders, a Nova Scotia shipbuilder to captain his schooner, the *Clotilda*, on a secret mission.[13]

The ship landed in Ouidah on the West Coast of Africa, (one of the transatlantic slave trading ports now in Benin) and exchanged $9,000 in gold and some rum for 110 persons in the holding pens or barracoons. In her posthumously published book, *Barracoon*, Zora Neale Hurston captured the recollections in the dialect of one of the last survivors of the horror, Cudjoe Lewis. Only nineteen when his village was raided, he could still recall all the brutal details. "I see de people gittee kill so fast! De old ones dey try run 'way from de house but dey dead by the door and de women soldiers got de head." The heads of his neighbors came to smell days after their decapitation and the stench followed them as their guards carried them on pikes. The king of Dahomey's military forces, who all transatlantic slavers visiting Ouidah were dependent upon, included a detachment of female soldiers, "Dahomey Amazons," who took part in raids of the interior to capture victims for the slave trade. It was the major source of income for the regime. Lewis recalled vividly his inspection by Captain Foster in the "Barracoon" or holding pen: "De white man lookee and lookee. He lookee hard at the skin and de feet and de legs and in de mouth. Den he choose."[14] Those chosen by Foster all managed to survive the Middle Passage to Mobile. Upon arrival, the *Clotilda* was burned and sunk to avoid any incriminating evidence. Federal charges against the participants in this scheme that hardly escaped notice in Mobile were dropped, because of the lack of physical evidence and the outbreak of the Civil War in 1861. The enslaved persons in the cargo were divided among the partners in the scheme but released from slavery by the arrival of US Army troops that included Black regiments at the end of the Civil War in 1865.

Free but lacking resources to return to their homeland, Lewis unsuccessfully argued with his former enslavers that they owed their formerly enslaved persons for the free labor provided in the past while enslaved and should compensate them with land. They scraped together some money on their own to buy some marginal land. The remaining enslaved cargo of the *Clotilda* set up "Africatown," their own hard scrabble community outside of Mobile, preserving their native language and other customs. Africatown's church, graveyard and some of its descendants are still in the area which is now on the register of national historic places. Cudjoe Lewis, the last survivor of the of the *Clotilda*'s final voyage, died in Africatown in 1935.

Archeologists found and confirmed the burnt submerged hulk of the *Clotilda* in 2019.[15]

The opening of rich land in Alabama and Mississippi for large scale cotton production made the purchase of enslaved persons profitable at almost any price. The cost of the enslaved persons and the land could be mostly recovered with a single crop. Using the purchased land and slaves as collateral, more land and enslaved persons could be acquired. It was an agri-industrial model that would not be matched elsewhere in the United States until the end of the twentieth century. There were large, short-term profits with higher risks of indebtedness and the dubious long-term sustainability of the single crop agricultural model. The massive investment in slavery, concentrated in Alabama and a few other deep south states, made peaceful elimination of slavery almost impossible. Slavery became the engine driving the rapid growth of the national economy, not the relic of an archaic order that would just pass with time. Emancipation in 1865 finally freed four million enslaved persons valued at an estimated fourteen billion in 2020 dollars.[16]

The agribusiness slave economy shaped Alabama and the American brand of capitalism. The demand for cotton in the textile mills in New England and England seemed to promise the Alabama plantations unlimited future wealth. Less than a quarter of white Alabama households owned enslaved persons, but that ownership shaped all aspects of life in Alabama. Enslaved persons were leased in the off season by their owners for construction of the railroads, bridges, and buildings in towns, helping to depress wages of white laborers and craftsmen. Bank capital tied up in loans to plantation owners for land and enslaved persons limited the opportunities to invest in economic diversification and better schools and other services. Some have argued that slavery was built into the genetic code of American capitalism, a low road that distinguished it from the one followed by most other capitalist democracies that included a much stronger role for labor unions and public sector social welfare investments.[17] The link between the methods used to increase enslaved person productivity on cotton plantations described by Rosenthal prior to the Civil War and the "scientific management" techniques of the progressive era embraced by industrialists for improving the productivity of their largely immigrant workforces is straight forward.[18]

Slavery transformed Alabama from a roughhewn democratic frontier culture into an autocratic police state in a few years. Anything that might threaten the institution of slavery was suppressed. Circulating or even having abolitionist literature was a crime punishable by flogging and imprisonment. Teaching enslaved persons to read or even allowing them to worship unsupervised became crimes. There was no such thing as a "free" press. The local press either suppressed anything that might question slavery, or they were run out of town. Local papers became active participants in the slave trade. Since the sale of enslaved persons often reflected the possibility of looming bankruptcy, owners preferred to preserve their anonymity and the newspapers helped manage slave transactions. Local newspapers also took part in organizing the entire white community in the capture of runaways and the punishment of those that helped them. They blurred the boundaries between private white vigilante actions and the law. Some would go on to fan the flames of mob violence during the upsurge in lynching in the early part of the twentieth century.

Only their rising value as property partially protected Alabama's enslaved from more brutal conditions. Plantation owners sought the help of physicians in Mobile to keep their enslaved persons healthy and productive. Influential Mobile physician Josiah Nott opened a clinic for the care of enslaved persons. Nott also, however, worked as a consultant estimating the price of life insurance policies on the enslaved. Such policies changed the calculations of slave owners whose asset was now protected but not the life of the enslaved person who could be hired out for risky mining and construction projects. Companies offering such policies included large northern ones such as New York Life, Aetna, and US Life, a subsidiary of American International Group (AIG), all of which still exist. New York Life sold 508 such policies in three years but the death claims in current dollars, about $232,000, almost matched its annual payments on the policies. Northern banks such as JP Morgan, Chase, and Wells Fargo allowed southerners to use the enslaved as collateral for loans, taking possession of them when their owners defaulted. Revelations of these past practices have produced recent embarrassment for these companies, as has state legislation insisting on a fuller and more accurate accounting of such past practices.[19]

Antebellum Mobile functioned like today's affluent gated winter resorts in Florida and along the Gulf Coast.[20] With a rapidly growing population of 29,258 in 1860, Mobile was the largest city in Alabama, and the center of a thriving cultural and social scene in winter months. Yellow fever epidemics emptied it out in the summer, but as a winter destination it offered white owners and their families respite from the isolation of plantation life. A theater, constructed in 1824, offered the first performance of Macbeth in Alabama in 1826. Concerts and ballets were also performed, along with Black-faced minstrel shows, jugglers, and trained animal acts. Pre-Lenten carnivals celebrated by mystic societies of Mobile's French and Spanish past were revived in the 1830s. The Battle House, a four-story luxury hotel completed in 1852, attracted plantation owner honeymooners and foreign visitors. Even a salon society modeled after the one in Paris became a part of the winter social scene. Madam Octavia Walton Leveret, a writer and wife of a prominent physician held an open house for the fashionable every Monday.[21]

As comforting as such amenities were for affluent planters and their families, the violence of a frontier port town lay just below the surface. Among the white aristocracy, too-close identification with the romantic novels of Sir Walter Scott about nobility could translate into duels of honor for insults on the edge of this fashionable winter social scene. A few blocks away by the wharfs, Bowie knife fights and eye gouging would break out among those lacking such aristocratic pretensions. Gambling, drinking, raucous dancing, and prostitution, just as in any frontier port town, flourished among all social classes.

Yellow fever, however, continued to wreak havoc in Mobile. Major epidemics took place in 1819, 1837 and 1839. During the 1839 one, Mobile men organized a "Can't Get Away Club" to raise funds for victims and set up a temporary hospital in a hotel for their care. The 1854 yellow fever killed 10 percent of Mobile's summer population. The severity of the epidemics, however, helped break caste barriers. For example, Pierre Chastang, an enslaved person, cared for and helped bury the Mobile victims of yellow fever in 1819. He was freed in recognition for these services and died in 1848 described as a "highly respected and esteemed member of the community."[22] In the wake of the COVID-19 pandemic something similar could happen.

Mobile's peculiar history also helped blur caste lines. In 1860, 41 percent of free Black citizens in Alabama resided in Mobile.[23] These included the Creoles descended from Spanish and French immigrants siring children with Black enslaved persons later freed under Spanish and French laws. Their rights were protected in the agreements leading to the Louisiana and North Florida acquisitions. Migrating freed enslaved persons seeking more opportunities added to the racial mix in Mobile. Free Black people in Mobile included prosperous merchants, barbers, blacksmiths, and carpenters. Some owned enslaved persons, with several owning as many as thirty.[24] Fearing the influence free Black residents might have on enslaved persons, both Mobile and the state of Alabama passed laws restricting interactions. For example, free Blacks had to follow an evening curfew and were prohibited from owning or operating bars, but Creoles were not. Alabama law in 1860 outlawed manumission as regional tensions increased.[25] The abundant diversity of skin colors and history would later make the enforcement of Jim Crow ordinances cumbersome.

The Catholic Church, supported by both the French and Spanish occupation of Mobile, stayed an influential force. Bishop Michael Portier constructed the Cathedral of the Immaculate Conception and founded Spring Hill College in 1833. Spring Hill would become a force in the racial desegregation of Mobile during the civil rights era. The Sisters of Charity managed the city hospital under contract beginning in 1852. The bishop also set up the Parish of St. Vincent De-Paul in 1847 to serve the Irish Catholic immigrants, who would soon supplant the Creole population as Mobile's largest Catholic ethnic group. The Irish Potato Famine (1844–1848) propelled that growth. In devastation, it could certainly qualify as a pandemic. About one million Irish died of starvation and another million emigrated. In 1860 about 24 percent of Mobile was foreign born and the Irish as for the largest group. Most of the Protestant churches, such as the Mobile Presbyterian Greek Revival church on Government Street, were constructed with the support of wealthy recent Northern settlers seeking business opportunities. Support for the institution of slavery was more ambivalent than in the rest of Alabama.

Mobile's cotton-slave economy faced increasing pressure from an anti-slavery world closing in around it. Almost all the northern states had enacted laws to phase out or outlaw slavery by the time the transatlantic slave trade was nationally outlawed in 1807. Britain abolished slavery in all its colonies except India in 1833 and the French followed in all its own colonies in 1848, both enforcing the ban on the transatlantic slave trade. A growing international abolitionist movement concentrated its focus on the Southern slave states. Abolitionist societies in the North grew in membership intent on freeing enslaved persons in the South. Slavery in the border states shrank as they shifted away from cotton to crops where the high cost of enslaved labor no longer made sense. Border state slave holders were selling many of their enslaved persons at good prices in the hard-core slave markets of the Deep South, such as Mobile.

Civil War

Mobile, as the rest of the nation, was ill prepared and ambivalent about the impending conflict. Dependent on the import of manufactured goods from northern or foreign industries and the export of cotton in exchange, Alabama's only major port could be easily blockaded. The rest of Alabama was not that unified by the Confederate cause either. About 100,000 Alabama men joined the Confederate forces, and 2,700 joined the Union Army, as did approximately 10,000 Black soldiers from the state.[26]

If Mobile and the rest of the nation had been unprepared for war, it was even more unprepared for its casualties. Four years later, at a cost of at least 625,000 American dead, about two thirds from disease, the insurrection ended. No other wars and only the influenza pandemic of 1918 and the COVID-19 pandemic of 2020 come close to its cost in American lives. Mobile did the best it could in caring for its share of the casualties. The Sisters of Charity used the City Hospital and Providence Hospital, a seventy-four-bed private Catholic one. Both cared for wounded Confederate soldiers, as did other hospitals in Alabama run by the order. They smuggled essential medical supplies from Union-occupied New Orleans.

Several Mobile women distinguished themselves aiding and organizing Confederate field hospitals. Juliet Hopkins volunteered and organized hospitals for Alabama soldiers in Virginia with donations from the relatives of the soldiers and Mobile residents. She was wounded twice retrieving harmed soldiers from the battlefield at Seven Pines near Richmond. Hopkins was later honored with her portrait engraved on two denominations of Alabama Confederate currency. Kate Cummings organized twenty-four other Mobile women to volunteer to care for Confederate soldiers wounded at the Battle of Shiloh in Southwestern Tennessee on April 6–7, 1862. Confederate losses included 1,728 dead and 9,012 wounded.[27] Grant later observed, "I saw an open field, in our possession on the second day, over which Confederates had made repeated charges the day before, so covered with the dead that it would have been possible to walk across the clearing in any direction, stepping on dead bodies, without a foot touching the ground.[28] Shiloh marked the beginning of an unwinnable war of attrition.

No Mobile figure cast a longer shadow over the Confederate cause and the development of medicine in the nineteenth century than Josiah Clark Nott. A Mobile surgeon, he stayed a steely supporter of white supremacy until his death after the War and Reconstruction had ended. In 1850 he owned sixteen enslaved persons. He also set up the J.C. Nott Infirmary in Mobile to treat free and enslaved Black residents. In addition, he consulted with life insurance companies, in helping to set prices that planters would have to pay to protect their slave assets. His family paid the ultimate price for his care of Mobile yellow fever victims and support of the war effort. Of his eight children, five died of yellow fever and two as soldiers in the Confederate cause. During the war, he served as a medical director of Confederate field hospitals.

Nott was Mobile's most influential medical leader. He had completed his medical degree at the University of Pennsylvania in Philadelphia and then interned at the Philadelphia Almshouse ("Old Blockley," or what would become Philadelphia General Hospital). Samuel Morton, a Penn professor of anatomy, served as an early mentor. Morton argued that the races had separate origins and that the white race was inherently superior. He amassed the largest collection of skulls in the world and used measurements of them to "scientifically prove" it. Upon Morton's death in 1852, Nott became the principal spokesperson for what was described as the "American School of Anthropology." The *Charleston Medical Journal* acknowledged Morton after his death, noting that "We can only say that we in the South should consider him our benefactor in giving the negro his true position as an inferior race."[29] Nott's position was the same.

The University of Pennsylvania is now in possession of Morton's collection of about 1,000 skulls.[30] It faces the unenviable task of respectfully returning them to their rightful communities. That would presumably include negotiations with the Cuban and West African governments.[31]

In addition to Nott's role, inherited from Morton, as the spokesperson for the American School of Anthropology, he devoted most of his career to medicine in Mobile. He helped create the Mobile Medical Society and the Alabama state medical society. He also helped found the Mobile Medical College and got the state legislature to supply the funding to construct a building to house it. It was later moved and renamed the University of Alabama School of Medicine.

Widely published and recognized as a medical leader of "scientific racism," Nott's reputation has became tarnished over time. As one twentieth century anthropologist saw, "Nott was less interested in the science of anthropology per se than he was in using selected portions of it to justify the continuation of special privileges for the white population in the antebellum South. At bottom, Nott was a prototypical Southern racist." His indignant correspondence with the superintendent of the Freedmen's Bureau, Major General O. Howard, who was in the process of requisitioning his medical school building for the education of the newly emancipated, was one of Nott's last intemperate salvos, "History proves indisputably that a superior and inferior race cannot live together practically on any other terms than master and slave, and that the inferior race, like the Indians, must be expelled or exterminated."[32]

Nott left Mobile soon after Reconstruction devastated his world. He set up a profitable obstetrics and gynecology practice in New York City. Nott survived Mobile's yellow fever epidemics, only to return shortly before his death at sixty-nine in 1878, after getting tuberculosis in New York City. No longer comfortable with his legacy, the Board of Trustees for University of Alabama's Tuscaloosa campus removed his name from a building that honored his role in August 2020.

Despite Nott's commitment to the Confederate cause, many in Mobile never shared it. Many just kept silent while others celebrated the State of Alabama's secession in January 1861, parading down Government Street to the Customs House to the tune of the La Marseillaise. Just as in the French Revolution, they marched to the same tune for different reasons.[33] Some supported radical white democracy and equality, while others a conservative return to aristocratic control. The differences surfaced first in arguments over a proposal to restrict suffrage of recent immigrants, mostly Irish. The White supremacy appeal for unity promised that Black residents would always occupy a position beneath them but left unresolved how power would be shared among them. Little has changed since then, except for the replacement of the Democratic party label for the Republican one.

Only when the parades and speeches ended, and the real costs of the conflict became clearer did the lack of support in Mobile become obvious. The city had difficulty getting help for construction of its defenses against Union forces.[34] Calls for volunteer help with their construction got little response. White Mobile residents regarded it as the kind of work that should only be done by enslaved persons. Slave owners resisted volunteering their enslaved people for such assignments and complained about their treatment by their Confederate overseers. When city officials proposed as an alternative a voluntary tax for raising funds for strengthening the City's defenses, it was opposed. Accusations of extortion and profiteering became common in 1862 and demands for government price controls grew. Farmers were accused of hording their crops until prices rose even further and the fishermen of dumping the catches to get higher prices. In September 1863 women took to the streets to protest merchant price gouging demanding "bread and peace," breaking into stores and stealing food and clothing. General Dabney H. Maurey, commander of District of the Gulf, ordered troops to stop the looting but they refused.[35] Suspicion fueled by the stark disparities in wealth overwhelmed more realistic assessments of the difficulties faced by the Union blockade. One woman blamed the "extortioners" as those who took "pleasure in the comforts and luxuries procured from heart's blood of the dying soldier, the tears of the needy widow and the dry crust that would hush the wail of a starving orphan."[36] Getting drunk legally, the local paper noted, was a mark of great wealth and status, because "a bottle of whisky could run several thousand Confederate dollars.[37] In 1863 the Confederate government received as much scorn as the private free market extortionists. As the war dragged on, morale in Mobile reached new lows. The local paper complained about the growing ambivalence to the war and open hostility toward the Confederate government. The major threat it argued came not from the Yankee invaders but from the apathy of people and their weariness. Many would not volunteer for military services or send their sons. Desertion rates rose and the boys were welcomed home instead of being ostracized. Surgeons freely gave out certificates of disability. As depravation spread, incidents of burglaries, receiving stolen goods, and illegal whisky-making increased. Further sacrifice seemed futile by mid-1864 when Admiral Farragut's fleet entered the Bay and Mobile prepared for an attack by Union troops.

In the last months of the war, while most in Mobile struggled to get food, some of its more affluent residents engaged in one last fling of parties in a world that would soon disappear. Lee surrendered to Grant at Appomattox on April 9, 1865. Mobile's mayor, accompanied by city dignitaries that included Dr. Nott, surrendered the city to the Union troops three days later.[38]

Snatching Victory from Defeat

Mobile's Reconstruction Era, as in the rest of the devastated Confederacy, was a violent roller coaster ride. In the first few months, about 136 Black persons in Mobile County were slaughtered by white mobs seeking revenge.[39] As described in Chapter 3, that ride continued in the twentieth century with Reconstruction Era lost cause myths contributing repeatedly to the death of national efforts to provide for universal health care.

In Mobile, the Reconstruction Era resolved nothing. It began with attempting to reestablish the old order, rose on the hopes of creating a new fairer one and then fell back into the old one. In the end, it left the condition of Black life little changed and left the Confederate lost cause narrative in defense of the old social order uncontested. Yet, Black resistance persisted.

Surrender in 1865 brought Union army occupation. Andrew Johnson assumed the presidency after Lincoln's assassination on April 15, 1865. He resisted enfranchisement of freedmen: "This is a government of white men and by God, as long as I am President it shall be a government of white men" he wrote to the governor of Missouri.[40] Alabama did a minor redrafting of Alabama's Confederate constitution prohibiting, at least on paper, slavery. The revised 1865 version of the constitution prohibited slavery but "It shall be the duty of the General Assembly, at its next session, and from time to time thereafter, to enact such laws as will protect the Freedmen of this State in the full enjoyment of all their rights of person and property, and guard them and the State against any evils that may arise from their sudden emancipation."[41] The first order of business for this "new" legislature, with the same leadership as the old Confederate one, was to develop a "Black Code," like ones developed in other former Confederate states, to assure that no such "evils" arose. One law in this code required adult males to enter labor contracts or supply other proof of employment. Those unable to do so could be convicted of vagrancy. Local law enforcement officials could then hire out these "vagrants" as contract laborers. This reimposed slavery—while never mentioning race. It remained in place in Alabama and other former Confederate states until World War II.[42] An "apprentice" law was also passed that allowed for orphans or children whose parents "refused" to support them to be put in the custody of a suitable person to serve an apprenticeship until adulthood. Such custody for former enslaved persons would typically go to their earlier masters. The threats of forced labor and confiscation of one's children served as powerful tools in reinforcing white supremacy. The laws never mentioned race, but everyone understood their intent. One legacy of this past is high incarceration rates. According to some sources, the United States has the largest incarcerated population and the highest incarceration rate of any nation in the world. That incarcerated population, while recently declining, still, includes more than two million persons, tenfold the total in 1972.[43]

Mobile, as Alabama's largest city, managed much of this transition from slavery to incarceration. It dealt with a large influx of former enslaved persons seeking food and employment. Local Black Code enforcement required all those violators to perform "labor for the benefit of the city as the mayor and the joint police council shall prescribe."[44] For this purpose, the Mobile police arrested Black loafers, idlers, and paupers. In addition, the freedmen newcomers were often attacked by white mobs concerned about their growing presence in the city. Black victims in these altercations would typically be the ones arrested. Irish immigrants concerned about their own job security were typically the perpetrators, but so was much of the Mobile police force. Alabama laws and customs also had never allowed Black people to testify in their own defense in court. The arrested Black victims would thus become participants in the contract (slave) labor system that was supposed to generate income for the city. Indeed, similar "color blind" contract labor arrangements still exist in the many Southern county criminal justice jurisdictions.[45]

The Mobile police force's handling of vagrancy and unruly behavior kept reasonable order with little of the vigilante terror that sprung up elsewhere in more rural Alabama. The Ku Klux Klan (KKK), founded in 1866 in neighboring Tennessee, spread quickly to rural areas of Alabama. The KKK targeted resistant Black organizers, federal Freedman's Bureau officials, and teachers in Black schools set up by Northern church groups with threats, whippings, and murders. Their effectiveness in sowing intimidation among Black Republican voters, however, led to unwanted Northern attention. The passage of the Ku Klux Klan Act in 1871 enabled president Ulysses S. Grant to use federal troops against the Klan and prosecute them in federal courts with predominantly Black juries. The Klan soon ceased to exist, only to resurface in 1915 long after federal oversight of Confederate states had ended.

The Northern voters, including many Union Army Veterans, gave the Republicans overwhelming control of Congress after the 1866 midterm elections. Congress overrode Johnson's veto of the Civil Rights Act of 1866, later ratified as the Fourteenth Amendment, which defined every person, regardless of race, born or naturalized in the United State as citizens with equal rights including the right to testify in court, own property, and be treated equally under the law. Congress went ahead to pass four Reconstruction Acts over Johnson's veto and then in 1868 to impeach him. They failed by only one vote to get the two-thirds majority needed to convict him in the Senate. Johnson still has the presidential record of veto overrides (15) but, in contrast to Trump, only one impeachment.

The four Reconstruction Acts in 1867 spelled out the guidelines for how federally controlled reconstruction would proceed over the next decade. The Act divided the ten "unreconstructed" states into five military districts commanded by Generals. Alabama and Mobile were part of the Third District that included Georgia and Florida. Former Confederate leaders would be ineligible to vote but freedmen were. Their first exercise of the franchise came with electing delegates to a new Alabama constitutional convention. Once the new constitution was approved by the electorate, with the same voting eligibility requirements in the Fifteenth Amendment that gave all male citizens the right to vote, regardless of race or earlier condition of servitude, the US Congress would then decide if Alabama was entitled to representation in Washington.

The Freedman's Bureau, set up by Lincoln before his death in 1865, became a division of his military command. They managed assistance to freedmen in buying food, housing, health care, education, and either finding employment or providing farmland. General Oliver Otis Howard served as Commissioner of the Freedman's Bureau. As part of his responsibilities, he founded Howard University. A century later, faculty in its law school and medical school would supply the key leadership for legal and medical Civil Rights reforms.

Most of the Bureau's staff were former Union soldiers. That Bureau's responsibilities for Alabama and Mobile fell to Assistant Commissioner General Wager Swayne. Swayne, trained as a lawyer, assumed this responsibility in August 1865 while still recovering from a combat leg amputation.[46] Swayne helped cut through state resistance and ordered all Alabama judicial officers to be considered Bureau agents, who would try cases involving Black residents no differently than white cases. If a local judge refused or continued to deny equal justice, he would lose his bureau appointment and martial law would be declared in his district. Lacking the staffing for direct bureau oversight, it was, however, a symbolic gesture. Even if Black people were allowed to testify, there was no assurance that the outcome would be any different.

In Mobile, when Swayne ordered the city's courts to allow Black citizens to testify, the mayor refused and resigned. Swayne replaced him with a mayor who would comply. Swayne also took over Josiah Nott's medical clinic and the Mobile Medical School building Nott had been the prime mover in creating. Swayne converted the medical school building into the Emerson School for Black children. The American Missionary Society assumed responsibility for their instruction. Enraged, Nott argued that children of the inferior Black race were not capable of receiving help from such formal education and that it would be a waste. Its creation served as a pointed symbolic refutation. Independent African American churches also sprang up in Mobile as educational resources. By 1868, about 800 Black children attended these sectarian schools in Mobile.[47]

Despite these efforts, Swayne was limited in completing the transformation of Mobile that radical reconstruction envisioned. Mobile continued to enforce its vagrancy ordinance on Black residents and, while never mentioning race, restricting Black workers to menial and lower paid employment. For example, hauling materials in the port on flatbed carts pulled by either mules or horses was a well-paid form of employment. The city approved an ordinance requiring a bond of $1,000 for such "drayman" to protect the purchaser of these services. These were available only to white draymen. The Black drayman's association protested to the Freedman's Bureau. The Bureau persuaded the city to reduce the bonds to $500, but this failed to eliminate the white drayman monopoly.[48]

Central to the radical reconstruction strategy was the extension of suffrage to Black males as passed in the 1867 Reconstruction Act.

Republicans in Mobile organized a Union League to serve as the organizing base for the Black electorate. Its leadership was biracial, including two white lawyers, the Black publisher of the *Mobile Nationalists*, and the minister of the African Methodist Episcopal Zion Church. The League's membership, growing to as many as 2,500, was almost all freedmen attracted by the promise of "security and protection of political rights and privileges."[49]

Democratic party leaders in Mobile responded both with appeals to "moderation" and threats. They campaigned to win support of the conservative and well-off Creole residents, who figured prominently in a public meeting organized by the mayor to discuss the new "political realities." The leaders urged that citizens work for "harmony and accord between the races" that was threatened by the Republicans. Freedmen, the Mayor argued, would receive nothing but trouble from the "radical Union League" and they should accept the leadership of the conservative white and Black coalition. In the meantime, employers in the city began a campaign to fire any Black workers suspected of joining the Union League. The all-white police department continued to harass Black citizens on the streets. Black dockworkers struck for higher wages with the encouragement of the Union League and were replaced with white workers. When the Black dockworkers tried to block the white ones from taking their jobs, the white Mobile police department prevented them.

Even so, freedmen pressed on, insisting that Black people had the right to ride on the city's streetcars. This provoked a brawl and the arrest of the leaders of the protest. Brigadier General Wager Swayne of the Freedmen's Bureau was able to broker a "compromise" with the streetcar company that allowed Black residents to ride in separate Black-only "Star Cars," Swayne also tried to end the practice of "apprenticing" Black minors to plantations and curb the enforcement of the vagrancy laws.

Threats of mob violence against Black people in Alabama and

the Republican Reconstruction effort soon became real. The Mobile Union League helped in registering Black men to vote and promoting their allegiance to the Republican Party. The local newspaper warned that retribution would come if the Union League continued "trading in the passions of an untutored race" and sowing "the seeds of a bloody war under the windows of the domestic hearth that enshrine our wives and daughters."[50] Indeed, the feared violence did come during a speech at a Union League gathering by visiting Congressman William D. "Pig Iron" Kelley (R, PA). He snapped back at white hecklers, reminding them that the US Army would protect his right to free speech. Shots were fired and a melee ensued. One Black and one white member of the audience were killed, and ten others wounded. The military authorities concluded that the local police had failed to supply adequate protection and ordered the mayor, the police chief, and the top city officials removed from office.

The Congressional Radical Republican Reconstruction plan went ahead with a state constitutional convention in 1867. Mobile's three Republican representatives included a recent white arrival from Maine, a former enslaved person now assistant editor of the city's Black newspaper, and a Creole assistant police chief. The new constitution heighted the racial fears of white Democrats and the hopes of Mobile's freedmen. It blocked a provision prohibiting interracial marriage, supported the racial integration of public schools, and endorsed suffrage for Black males. The later-elected state legislature ratified the Fourteenth Amendment guaranteeing citizenship to all persons, including former enslaved persons, born or naturalized in the United States, and guaranteed all citizens "equal protection under its laws." In 1868 Alabama regained representation in the US Congress. The delegation included two Republican senators who had served as Union soldiers and five Republicans in the six-man House delegation. Four of these had been Freedman's Bureau Agents, one was a freedmen and only one was a long-time Alabama resident.

Furious, white Mobile natives continued to resist. The abolitionist fervor in the North that had fueled the radical Republican
reconstruction plan waned as the cost of military occupation of the
Confederate states mounted. Reconstruction was the nineteenth-
century equivalent of the recently ended occupation of Afghanistan,
with a similar, inevitable outcome. The local election in Mobile in
1874 and the national presidential one in 1876 ended all hopes of real
reconstruction for almost a century. The freedmen that Republican
Reconstruction had tried to protect suffered the consequences.

Mobile politics during reconstruction until the 1874 election offered at least a little room for compromise. "Radical" Republicans
argued for full integration of public services such as street cars
and schools. The "Old South" Democrats, bristled at any gestures
that hinted at undermining white supremacy. More "moderate" Republicans and Democrats, however, could still forge alliances that
acknowledged Black suffrage and cultivated their votes, while not
violating informal norms of racial separation. For example, a Republican mayor advocated spending cuts, a trademark of Democratic political candidates, and closed the city soup kitchen, alienating much
of his Black Republican constituency. Democratic leaders supported
the reelection of a mayor who supported their plan for development
of the port. They also gained support from Black Republicans by not
interfering in a successful Black dock worker strike in 1870 and supporting the shift to better access for Blacks to the city's street cars.

In the 1874 city elections Democrats, however, returned to power
replacing Black police officers with white ones and cutting social services. The middle ground disappeared. Groups called White Men's
Associations organized throughout the city, seething with racial and
class resentments raised to a fever pitch by proposals of the Republicans to integrate the public schools. The 8th Ward White Men's
Association declared, "Whites must answer to the call of white supremacy over the black monkey mimics of civilization, who arrogate

superiority over men whom God made their masters, not in chattel slavery of their persons, but to dominate them in intellect, in morals and in native worth."[51] They swore to battle the Republican "radicals" who sought the "annihilation of the prosperity of the South, the degradation of her people and the utter destruction of her distinct independent national identity" through the manipulation of "former barbarian slaves."[52]

During the election, armed gangs roamed the streets threatening Black voters at gunpoint. Mobs gathered around polling places blocking all but Democratic sympathizers from voting. Ballot boxes were stuffed, and counts were altered by Democrats. Yet, the cost of invalidating the election from the perspective of the Union oversight just seemed too high. The Democrats won. A volatile white supremacy coalition joined the white elite to the white working class. They shared little else in common but would dominate Mobile politics for a century. Reconstruction, as far as Mobile was concerned, was over.

Nationally, reconstruction ended with an even more bitterly contested national Presidential election in 1876. Republican Rutherford B. Hayes and Democrat Samuel J. Tilden fought to a stalemate resolved by a Congressional electoral commission. That "precedent" was revisited again in a proposal by some Republican members of congress in 2021, questioning the validity of the Biden win. Victory in 1876 hinged on disputed results from three Confederate states still occupied by federal troops (South Carolina, Florida, and Louisiana). The Black Republican vote had been suppressed by violence and intimidation just as it had earlier in the 1874 Mobile City election. The Commission created by Congress gave the election to Hayes. An informal "compromise," however, made that victory a costly one. Never put in writing and with the threat of a renewal of the Civil War in the air, it exchanged the presidency for Hayes for the removal of all remaining troops from the Confederacy and a return to state "home rule." It put an end to federal reconstruction efforts and any Black electoral influence in the South.

How the Lost Cause Myth Reigned Supreme

During the 1946 Nuremburg Trials war-crimes defendant Hermann Goering reportedly observed, "The victor will always be the judge, and the vanquished the accused." The US Civil War may be the only one that didn't work out that way. In essence, the Confederate states were left to manage their own affairs—arguably the cause for which they had fought. They also captured the national political narrative about Reconstruction that would dominate the Jim Crow era and beyond. How did the "vanquished" end up serving as the judge and the "victor" the accused? For the Confederate South, 1877 heralded the beginning of "Redemption." That meant being saved from evil and a return to uncontested white supremacy. In the symbolism of current politics, it would have included lots of people at rallies wearing MCGA (Make the Confederacy Great Again) hats in lieu of the Trump MAGA ones. Redemption required two things: (1) the acceptance of a myth culled from selective memories of Reconstruction that would justify white supremacy, and (2) the creation of an institutional structure that would assure its permanence.

The fable of the vanquished about reconstruction went something like this: The War had been a "tragic mistake." The South had willingly accepted emancipation and Lincoln's plans for a quick and gracious accommodation that would have restored the Union. Instead, the Radical Republicans grasped control, seeking revenge, economic spoils, and political gain. Overriding vetoes by Lincoln's successor, Johnson, they imposed military rule, disenfranchising white citizens and enfranchising freedmen. The result was an era of corrupt and incompetent chaos. It ended when the states of the Confederacy finally wrestled home rule control back from the federal government and, peacefully or by force, from the freedmen and their carpetbagger and scalawag allies, assuring honest, competent government in the South under its natural leaders.

The fable appealed to the pride and resentment of white southerners of the federal intervention. No one wanted to accept responsibility for a disaster as catastrophic as the Civil War. The lost cause myth prevented this—they did not really lose; they were just tricked and cheated. It fit well with the Southern antebellum myth of an idyllic world ruled by genteel aristocrats who looked after their enslaved people with the same concern as family members, a "golden age." The lost cause myth includes all the romantic nostalgia of Mobile's own bestselling Civil War and Reconstruction Era novelist—Augusta Evans Wilson (1835–1909). Wilson, as we will soon see, has her fingerprints all over the struggle told in this book.

Why, however, was this fable accepted so easily by the Northern "victors"? The truth is that the racial views of white society in the North were not that different from those of white elites in the South. It was easy for white Northerners to oppose slavery since they did not have any enslaved persons. The hard core white radical Republicans and abolitionists committed to full racial equality were a minority. Most northern whites had a hard time accepting the idea of full racial integration and equal opportunity for better paying jobs. Weariness soon replaced pride in the Civil War victories. The treatment of Black people in states of the former Confederacy were just too distant from northern concerns.

As a result, the white Southerners had a monopoly in producing the official narrative surrounding Reconstruction. They had the home field advantage. Elaborate Southern antebellum myths in defense of slavery just needed a little elaboration. Josiah Clark Nott, MD, of Mobile had been an influential contributor to the white superiority antebellum literature that found widespread acceptance at Northern and European medical schools. Thomas Dixon Jr. and William

Archibald Dunning were two of the southern Reconstruction era "lost cause" myths most influential contributors.

Thomas Dixon Jr., born just before the end of the Civil War in North Carolina, grew up during Reconstruction. His father, a former slave owner, joined the Klan and an uncle, Colonel Leroy McAfee became its head, the "Grand Titan of the Invisible Empire Ku Klux Klan," in Piedmont, North Carolina. Dixon's childhood memories included bitterness over Reconstruction and hero worship of an uncle who took part in the town square lynching of a Black man accused of raping a white woman. Dixon later produced skillful white supremacy polemics in his lectures, sermons, romantic novels, films, and racist propaganda at the turn of the twentieth century. The books in his "Klan trilogy," *The Leopard's Spots: A Romance of the White Man's Burden 1865–1900* (1905), *The Klansman: A Historical Romance of the Ku Klux Klan* (1906), and *The Traitor: The Story of the Fall of the Invisible Empire* (1907), all became best sellers. They romanticized white supremacy, promoted the lost cause of the Confederacy, opposed equal rights for Black people, and glorified the Ku Klux Klan members as heroic vigilantes. The villains in Dixon's fiction were Black men who raped white women, and the heroes were the Klan vigilantes who exacted justice by lynching them.

Today it would be assumed that such material was the product of a marginal, unhinged, and dangerous extremist on an FBI watch list. It is hard to understand now how influential and mainstream Dixon was. After graduating from Wake Forrest, Dixon enrolled in the graduate program in Political Science at Johns Hopkins University where he befriended fellow student Woodrow Wilson. He was later offered an honorary doctorate at Wake Forrest but declined arguing that the honor should go to his friend at Hopkins, giving Wilson his first national exposure. Dixon rose to be pastor of the Twenty-Third Street Baptist Church in New York City, with the largest congregation of any Protestant church in the United States. He rubbed elbows with John D. Rockefeller and Theodore Roosevelt and campaigned for Roosevelt in his race for governor. As a widely acclaimed lecturer on the Chautauqua circuit, about five million attendees heard him speak over a four-year period. Dixon is best known for authoring *The Klansman*, which D. W. Griffith transformed into a movie, later renamed *The Birth of a Nation*. It was promoted by a showing at Wilson's White House. The movie helped stimulate the rebirth of the Klan.

The more academically respectable version of the lost cause myth, however, was generated by William Archibald Dunning, a history professor at Columbia University, and his like-minded students. A Southerner who grew up accepting the lost cause fable of Reconstruction, he and the students attracted to him from similar backgrounds fleshed out the myth with archival scholarship. Known as the "Dunning School" of Reconstruction history, they deplored the decade of federal intervention as the "tragic era of Negro misrule."[53] This characterization of the period dominated high school and college history textbooks in all regions of the country through the 1960s. The recent local and state conservative backlash against teaching so-called "critical race theory" in public institutions wants to return to the Dunning School.

Finally, any alternative narrative offered by Black voices was either silenced or coopted. Frederick Douglass, powerful voice of the abolitionist movement and despairing critic of its betrayal after 1877, died in 1895. A year later, Booker T. Washington captured center stage in Black national leadership with his "Atlanta Compromise" speech. More attuned to the realities facing Black people in the South, he proposed conceding to the white supremacy myth in exchange for support for peaceful but separate educational and economic development. Washington left the Southern white Reconstruction fable unchallenged, and even reinforced it. Founder of the Tuskegee Institute in Alabama, he worked magic in extracting money from both white and Black business leaders in pursuing his vison of separate Black development. W. E. B. Du Bois would succeed Washington as the most influential Black voice and would challenge Washington's accommodationist approach. In 1935 he published his major scholarly rebuttal, *Black Reconstruction in America*.[54] The work was ignored by white mainstream historians until the 1960s. Hounded by the FBI and McCarthyism in the 1950s, Du Bois spent the last two years of his life in exile in Ghana. He died in 1963 the day before the March on Washington, where he was honored with a moment of silence. At the March, Martin Luther King would give his "I have a Dream" speech in support of civil rights legislation that Du Bois had supported for half a century. It would pass a year later. The resistance movement would have a brief opportunity to change the narrative.

In Mobile, of course, the only possibility was to follow Booker T. Washington's accommodationist strategy. The presence of a large Creole population helped supply a model. Black residents accounted for about 40 percent of Mobile's population, and Black entrepreneurs succeeded in developing a practical parallel Black business community. From the 1870s onward, that community included three drug stores owned and run by a Black physician and a furniture manufacturing business that was the largest operated by Black laborers in Alabama. Although less prone to racial violence than rural areas in the South, it was hardly idyllic. With ratification of the 1901 Constitution, Black citizens disappeared from the voter registration rolls. A boycott of segregated trolley cars collapsed. In 1906, for the first time in Mobile County, a mob lynched two Black men accused of rape. A similar instance followed in the city. A Black man was taken from the county jail and lynched across the street in front of the city's oldest church.[55]

Black citizens became invisible as a political constituency in Mobile at the same time as the rise in lynching and the popularity of the works of Dixon and of the Dunning school. In 1905 President T. R.

Roosevelt visited the city. He refused to address a Black audience or even meet with Black leaders, despite their support for the Republican party. When President Woodrow Wilson later visited the city in 1913, Black residents were similarly ignored. These slights were representative of Progressive movement indifference to Black suffering and disenfranchisement in the Jim Crow era. The *Plessy v. Ferguson* decision in 1896, had given federal constitutional approval to Jim Crow. What had been informally evolving in Mobile since 1874 would soon be cast into concrete.

CHAPTER FIVE

Struggles with Jim Crow

JEAN COWSERT RETURNED TO HER hometown to set up a medical practice in 1959. Military service, undergraduate, medical school education, and an internship and residencies in Detroit had kept her away, except for brief visits, for almost eighteen years. Cowsert had changed but so had Mobile. It was no longer the nostalgic city of her childhood. The struggle with Jim Crow was coming to a head. Its two pillars, segregation and disenfranchisement, stood unyielding. She would be swept along, using all that she had learned in her absence, but unsure where it would take her. In doing so, she rubbed shoulders with four key local civil rights leaders. With limited resources, they faced off in a brutally bitter battle with four of Alabama's most powerful defenders of Jim Crow. Jean Cowsert joined in the medical side of this struggle. Most take the world they are born into and grow up in for granted. Like most, Jean Cowsert had little awareness of the difficulties this past would now pose for her.

Mobile's Jim Crow Cage

During the first decade of the twentieth century, Alabama and Mobile erected the two essential pillars of Jim Crow—racial segregation and disenfranchisement. Segregation imposed a caste order and disenfranchisement ended any voice in opposition to it. Alabama's 1901 constitution and Mobile's 1911 at-large commissioner form of government put an end to any Black voice. Solidly constructed, only after World War II did civil rights resistance begin to disassemble that cage.

Alabama functioned under its 1901 Constitution until 2022. As stated by John B. Knox, chairman of the Constitutional Convention, its purpose was to, "within the limits of the Federal Constitution, establish White supremacy in this state."[1] It was modeled after the Mississippi Constitution of 1890 that had survived a series of federal court challenges. To be eligible to vote, males had to pass a literacy test administered by local white officials. A "grandfather clause" exempted anyone who had served in the military or was descended from someone who had. This excluded Black males and their descendants since they were mostly excluded from military service. Females, "idiots and insane persons," persons who married interracially, and people who were convicted of a "crime against nature" (homosexuality) or vagrancy were also excluded. Younger-aged voters either needed to pay a cumulative yearly poll tax or, alternatively, own forty acres or other property assessed at more than $300 for which all taxes had been paid. This excluded the poor of all races. Indeed, by 1940 the 1901 Alabama Constitution had excluded more white residents from voting than Black.[2]

The 1901 Constitution was never intended to achieve greater "white democracy." Its purpose was to assure that a coalition of Black citizens, white Republicans, and populists (typically small farmers and blue-collar workers mostly from the northern part of the state) never gained control. White Democratic control was further assured by giving limited authority to the executive branch and giving representation to the more powerful legislative branch in favor of the state's more rural counties. All sixty-seven counties doubled as legislative districts. Each county elected one senator and at least one representative. County lower house representatives were supposed to be apportioned by population, but no reapportionment took place for sixty years. This not only violated the state constitution but grossly underrepresented growing urban areas such as Mobile. Federal court challenges in the 1960s tried to address this imbalance. The state legislature, however, even today still exercises inordinate control over local matters. Most of the tax code is written into the constitution. Even Mobile, which eventually gained limited home rule, had to get a constitutional amendment passed to implement a local mosquito control tax. Indeed, part of the persistent resistance to replacing the 1901 Constitution comes not from eliminating its remaining racist language but from a conservative visceral antipathy to any taxes and its success in blocking them.[3] Alabama taxes *increase* family after-tax income disparities. The state ranks as the eighteenth most regressive in the nation as well as thirty-eighth in spending per public school pupil.[4]

Most Alabama residents regarded its 1901 constitution an embarrassment. It prohibited interracial marriage and mandated racially segregated public schools. Federal court decisions have found that many of its provisions violate the Federal Constitution. Some of these provisions had led to cumbersome amendments and others had been left in with the informal understanding that they would not be enforced. One side effect of this effort to centralize control and limit support of local services is a constitution that includes more than 310,296 words, the longest and most amended constitutional document in the world.[5] A plan to remove some of its more embarrassing racist language and the incomprehensible organization of its local amendments was considered by the legislature in 2022. According to the chair of the legislative committee submitting the plan, "the document is supposed to reflect who we are in this state. We're black, we're white, we're Democrats, Republicans, we're rich, we're poor."[6] As a result of these efforts, Alabama voters finally approved a "new" constitution in November 2022. The Alabama Constitution of 2022 did a masterful editing job, shortening the text, removing racist language, improving organization, and generally making the 1901 document more readable. Other than these editing changes, voters were assured "the reorganized constitution will make no changes other than those listed above and will not make any changes relating to taxes."[7] Status quo for Blacks, whites, rich, poor, Democrats, and Republicans. Same body politic, just more presentable clothes. The earlier campaign for ratification of the 1901 Constitution included less presentable attire. It included the slogan "White Supremacy! Honest Elections! and the New Constitution! One and Inseparable!"[8] The vote supporting its passage appears to have been a victim of the fraud the new constitution was supposed to eliminate.[9] Not concerned with such subtleties, the front-page headline in the *Montgomery Advertiser* read: "The Citizens of Alabama Declare for White Supremacy and Purity of Ballot. The Putrid Sore of Negro Suffrage is Severed from the Body Politic of the Commonwealth. New Constitution Carries by a Majority that is Overwhelming."[10]

The 1901 Constitution preceded a similar change in Mobile governance. In 1911, Mobile changed from a Mayor-Council, with council members elected to local wards, to a three-member commissioner form, with the three commissioners elected at large. Black representation on city council previously came from a majority Black ward. The majority population of Mobile was white, so the reorganization succeeded in excluding any Black representation. The Mayor-Council structure returned only after a protracted series of court battles in 1985. The *Wiley Bolden v. City of Mobile* case hinged on proving the "intent" to discriminate. The smoking gun evidence of this came from an open letter written in 1909 by a strong advocate of the commissioner structure, US Congressman Fredrick Bromberg (D, AL) of Mobile, to the Alabama State Legislature reminding the legislators that "we have always, as you know, falsely pretended that our purpose was to exclude the ignorant vote, when, in fact, we were trying to exclude not the ignorant vote but the Negro vote."[11]

The Supreme Court decision in *Plessy v. Ferguson* in 1896, the White Supremacy Constitution of 1901, and the change to commission structure in Mobile in 1911 set the stage for a half century of Jim Crow. Black residents in Mobile still had political relevance up until the ratification of the 1901 Constitution.[12] No local chapter of the Klan existed. Mobile's white leaders could argue that, unlike other areas of the former Confederacy, there were no lynchings.[13]

Jim Crow changed Mobile. Segregation no longer had to rely on informal customs or subtle white intimidation. Mobile passed a city ordinance segregating streetcars, requiring Black riders to sit in the back. A two-month, Black-organized boycott collapsed. Two years later the City Council upheld the exclusion of Black community members from the oldest park in the city. Soon all public spaces and facilities in the city were either segregated or made white only. By 1913 Black people in Mobile lived in a separate and unequal world, born in separate settings, and buried in separate cemeteries. Notices of deaths and marriages in the *Mobile Register* appeared in separate columns. A local activist recalled, "To look in the classified section of the paper for a job was a nightmare. You had to remember not to look under 'Male and Female Help Wanted.' That was for white workers. Blacks were classified as 'domestic helpers'— you had to wait and see if it read "Colored." . . . The paper would read 'House for Sale.' You had to remember that this meant houses for whites only. Houses for Blacks were listed as 'Houses, Lots for.'"[14]

Jim Crow laws in Mobile exacerbated racial "friction" rather than ending it as some had argued. In its twentieth-century rebirth, Mobile claimed its first local chapter of the Klan, and by 1921, it had two thousand members.[15] Six lynchings took place in Mobile County between 1906 and 1919.

Two lynchings illustrate the unraveling of Mobile's reputation for racial moderation. In 1906, a twenty-year-old Black waiter named Will Thompson and Cornelius Robinson, a seventeen-year-old unemployed Black laborer, were both accused of raping young white girls. They were to be escorted out of town to avoid mob vengeance. With the assurance of state troops to protect them, the two prisoners were being transported back to Mobile by train for trial when forty-five masked white men with rifles boarded the train and captured the prisoners just outside Mobile. Despite appeals to let the legal process proceed, the two were strung up on a tall tree nearby. Repeating the grotesque scenes taking place elsewhere in the South, over three thousand morbid sightseers flocked to view the suspended bodies. The corpses were photographed to be sent as postcards. Fragments of the victims' clothing, ropes, and bark from the tree were taken as souvenirs.[16]

In January 1909, anti-Black violence was again on display in Mobile. Two deputies, Philip Fetch and W. N. McCarron, tried to serve a warrant on Richard Robertson, a mixed-race carpenter. Robertson opened fire with a .38 and all three were wounded in the ensuing gun battle. Fetch died that night in a hospital. During the early morning hours, thirty masked men carried the wounded Robertson from his cell at the county jail and hanged him from the large oak tree on the corner of Church and St. Emanuel streets—directly across from Christ Episcopal Church, the city's oldest place of worship. The sheriff and his deputies had neither locked the jail nor offered any resistance. While the lynching occurred within two blocks of central police headquarters in an affluent residential area where police officers walked regular beats, no officers appeared. Gazing out of her living-room window, a woman saw Robertson hanging from the tree and called the police. The officer on duty informed her that he knew the lynching was in progress.

Those raising questions about the affair got a threatening letter from an anonymous "Committee of 100" saying, "You and your friends are going to get a rope around your neck if you don't keep your mouth shut about that Negro lynching."[17] To the city reformers' credit, they did not. Since the threats were sent by the US postal service, they explored the possibility of prosecuting the perpetrators in federal court. In the end, because they could not find any witnesses willing to testify against the sheriff in the grand jury proceedings, they pursued impeachment of the sheriff in the state courts. In a five-to-two decision in June 1909 the Alabama Supreme Court ruled the Mobile sheriff was guilty of impeachable offenses and he was removed from office. It was a small, symbolic victory in grim times.

World War II

Mobile's Jim Crow structure, implemented in the first two decades of the twentieth century, remained unaltered for another two. The shock of World War II began to force change, but it took time. At a meeting of the Southern Historical Association in Memphis, in November 1982, Morton Soa of Stanford presented a paper suggesting that World War II had a more profound impact on the South than the Civil War. The commentator on the paper observed, only half in jest, "I felt obliged to warn him that while such radical notions might be tolerated or even encouraged at Stanford, it was quite another thing to stand at the northern terminus of the Mississippi Delta and dare suggest that any event in human history, save perhaps the birth and resurrection of Jesus Christ, was more important than the Civil War. To my surprise he not only delivered his paper but lived to see it published."[18]

In no place in the South did World War II have as profound an effect as in Mobile.[19] Defense industry expansion produced a 64 percent increase in the Mobile Metropolitan Area population during the four war years, surpassing Montgomery as Alabama's second largest city. Gulf Shipbuilding and Alabama Dry Dock and Shipping

Company (ADDSCO) sprung to life. Both poor rural white and Black workers flocked to Mobile seeking better-paying jobs. Gaps in income and wealth narrowed and the GI Bill offered new opportunities for job training, higher education, and home ownership. In 1940 only 7 percent of Alabamans had any education beyond high school. By 1950 those with some college education had increased to 43 percent. Agriculture ceased to dominate the economy of the region, becoming part of a more mixed sunbelt economy that was urban and suburban in character.

Mobile's Black population became more assertive as it grew from twenty-nine thousand in 1940 to forty-six thousand a decade later. Black residents threatened to boycott Mobile's bus system after a Black soldier was shot to death by a bus driver. The bus company averted the boycott by promising more courteous treatment and agreeing to disarm its drivers. The most racially tense incidents during the war years came when Mobile's Jim Crow challengers demanded the shipyards follow fair employment practices. In response, Alabama Dry Dock and Shipbuilding Company (ADDSCO) added twelve Black welders to an all-white night shift crew. As the news spread to the morning shift, white workers began assaulting Black ones. Injured Black laborers fled the work site. Troops from the Brookley Field Airbase restored order. A year later Black troops at Brookley Field opened fire on white military police who entered their segregated housing compound to investigate a robbery complaint.[20]

In May 1944 tensions rose again at the planned ship-launching ceremonies of the *Tule Canyon*. An all-Black construction crew had completed its assembly in record time and were to be singled out for praise. A rumor spread that resentful white workers would "clear the yard of all Negroes to prevent them from witnessing or participating in the launching."[21] ADDSCO officials responded by placing armed guards and planting more than one hundred informants in the crowd gathered to see the event. The earlier violence against Black workers was not repeated, and the *Tule Canyon* launch celebration went ahead without incident.

The Challengers and Defenders of Jim Crow

Even with the impact of World War II, the odds for those fighting Jim Crow were long and the risks high. The challengers in Mobile called attention to themselves and became targets. White Citizens Councils appeared after the *Brown* decision to better organize efforts to crush any challenger's ability to make a living. Few were insulated from such threats. Most paid their dues in cash to the local NAACP chapter and kept their membership secret. Few could be listed as plaintiffs in civil rights suits. Black public schoolteachers might be tolerated as registered voters, because if they got too "uppity" they could always be fired by the white school board. Only those totally insulated or segregated from local white control had any job protection. Only the names of Black ministers, doctors, dentists, and, in the case of Mobile, federal civil service post-office employees could appear on the letterhead of civil rights organizations or as plaintiffs in legal cases.

White Citizens Councils and more respectable middle class white supremacists in Mobile avoided engaging in physical violence but that threat, whether conducted by ad hoc faceless mobs or by a growing Klan presence in Mobile, was always there. Some Black Alabamans chose to join the Great Migration in hopes of greater safety in the North. Four Mobile residents never stopped challenging the Jim Crow status quo. They lacked the resources of its powerful defenders, but they never stopped trying. Mobile's civil rights story is best captured in the stories of those four challengers: John LeFlore, Albert Foley, Joseph Langan, and Noble Beasley.

John LeFlore (1903–1976), the fifth of five children, faced all of Mobile's predictable indignities of poverty and race. His father died before he was a year old, and his mother took in laundry to support the family. At five, John began to help by selling the *Mobile Press* newspaper. His first racial confrontation came from reading one of the papers he was selling. A white man caught him, snatched the paper away, threw it in the river, telling him n . . . . youngsters weren't supposed to be reading and that he better not catch him doing it again.[22] More discreetly he persisted, gaining a job at the local post office. Married in 1922, his honeymoon was marred because he and his wife were refused access to the Pullman dining car and sleeping accommodations on their trip to St. Louis.

The final straw for him came three years later. LeFlore, tired from a day of mail delivery, climbed on a Mobile trolley, taking the last seat available.[23] Several minutes later, a white man climbed on and demanded his seat. He would have voluntarily given up the seat unrequested if it had been a woman or a physically incapacitated person, but this individual was perfectly capable of standing and just felt entitled to the seat because of the color of his skin. The resulting argument degenerated into a fight. He was held at gunpoint by the trolley driver until a police officer arrived to arrest him for disorderly conduct. He spent the night in jail and had to produce $100 for bail. The officer let the white man go free. That was the beginning of LeFlore's life-long career as a civil rights activist.

LeFlore, as would become a habit, described in a detailed complaint the circumstances surrounding his arrest and sent it to the national office of the NAACP. This brought him an invitation to set up a chapter in Mobile. The first Mobile chapter, founded in 1919, had shut down when all of it members resigned because of white threats of retaliation. LeFlore took on the post of branch secretary for the new chapter in 1926. His livelihood as a federal civil service postal employee, while threatened, offered some protection. The other members of the new chapter shared similar employment protections that members of the original chapter had not. The new members included twelve postal workers, five life insurance agents, two dentists, two undertakers, and a physician, all serving Mobile's Black community and thus insulated from white retaliation.

For the next two decades, Mobile had the only active local NAACP chapter in Alabama. The case load included appealing a Black man's murder conviction as the result of a coerced confession. Closer to LeFlore's own experiences, the chapter's complaints led to eight interstate rail companies beginning to equalize the availability of restaurants and sleeping cars for Black passengers. In addition, the local chapter's pressure resulted in added jobs for Black postal workers.

LeFlore and the local chapter played a central role in finding resolutions to the explosive racial violence surrounding Mobile's shipbuilding growth during World War II. LeFlore focused mostly on "bread and butter" issues such as the training of Black welders for some of the higher paying jobs in the shipyards and an end to the discriminatory local practices in the licensing and inspection of Black beauticians. He and the local chapter also played a central role in the looming Black voter registration battles in Mobile.

LeFlore's early actions were neither timid nor passive. He investigated and reported to the National Office on lynchings taking place across the South. Between 1942 and 1952 he also served as a staff writer for the *Chicago Defender* and the *Pittsburgh Courier*, traveling alone to investigate such events and risking retaliation as an outside troublemaker. As a postal carrier, he did not share the relative economic security of the Black physicians and dentists who served in such local leadership capacities. For forty years he had to deal with the threat of being fired. White Mobile postal officials tried to apply the Hatch Act, which prohibits postal employees from engaging in partisan political activity. In 1935, the white Mobile postmaster argued that his work with the NAACP violated this prohibition and demanded LeFlore be fired. Only a strong letter of protest to the Postmaster General from the NAACP national office blocked this from happening. Thurgood Marshall as Special Counsel also had to write a strong protest letter in 1946 to block a similar attempt.

Nevertheless, LeFlore faced increasing local criticism in his role as secretary of the Mobile chapter of the NAACP after World War II. The rival Veterans and Voters Association criticized him for being too conservative in his approach. The local NAACP chapter faced a loss of membership because of its inability to deal with a rise in police violence and an upswing in Klan activity in Mobile. The chapter ceased to exist in 1956 after Judge Walter Jones of the State Circuit Court in Montgomery outlawed the NAACP in Alabama because of its refusal to make public its membership lists. LeFlore, however, adeptly shifted his activities to ones under the auspices of a local organization that he had helped form earlier, the Nonpartisan Voters League. The League named LeFlore to the position of director of casework. This enabled him to set its legal agenda and gave him a degree of local independence he had not had as an officer of the NAACP. In 1957 under his direction, the League began publishing a "Pink Sheet," a pamphlet circulated in Mobile's Black community that included a list of candidates considered supportive of the Black community's interests. The Black minority in Mobile could still sway the outcome between competing candidates in at-large elections for commissioners. The Nonpartisan Voter's league did not have to contend with the constraints against directly taking part in electoral politics imposed on the NAACP.

LeFlore was a force in the politics of Mobile until his death from a heart attack in January 1976. He played a central role in the efforts to desegregate Mobile's school system described later in this chapter and in the desegregation of Mobile's hospitals, which will be described in detail in the final section of this book. LeFlore believed in quiet negotiation, persuasion, and legal actions rather than street protests and would come under increasing criticism by more militant activists. The firebombing of his home in 1967 would suggest that none of his more violence-prone opponents regarded him as ir-relevant. His election to the state house in 1974 from Mobile where he served until his death suggested that most in Mobile still trusted his judgment.

Albert Foley Jr. (1912–1989) was born in New Orleans. He grew up in a segregated world that he and other white people took for granted. As a young boy, he attended a showing of the *Birth of a Nation* and found it "inspiring."[24] The Catholic Church of his faith took it all for granted as well. The Klan had a strong anti-Catholic streak and the South's Catholic Church hierarchy kept a low profile on racial issues. Change came after he had become a Jesuit priest and sociologist, when he was assigned to teach a course on "mi-gration, immigration, and race" at Spring Hill College in Mobile during the summer of 1943. He interviewed Black Catholics about their Jim Crow experiences, asked fundamental ethical questions, and started becoming an activist. The Mobile Bishop warned him to stay away from the issue of "social equality which leads to noth-ing but trouble" and, when that warning failed, arranged for Foley's reassignment.

Father Foley, however, returned in 1947 to Spring Hill to teach sociology and to spend the rest of his life there. He served as chair-person of the Mobile chapter of the Alabama Council on Human Re-lations, as well as the Alabama Advisory Committee to the United States Civil Rights Commission and worked closely with Martin Luther King Jr. He collaborated with John LeFlore and his NAACP chapter and Nonpartisan Voters League, as well as with Joseph Lan-gan, who would serve as a liberal City Commissioner.

Foley had a scrappier, more confrontational style than his other Mobile collaborators. In 1958 he authored two model city ordinances, one banning Mobile police department members from membership in the Klan and the other banning "intimidation by exhibit" (e.g., cross burning). Enraged, the local Klan ran an advertisement attacking him as "a man of large profession and small deeds, a communist and quisling of foreign seed who wants to write city ordinances."[25]

Since the FBI never responded to his request for Klan surveillance, he took on the job himself. Foley hired individuals to take down license plate numbers at Klan meetings and compile a list of local Klan members, and he employed others to infiltrate their meetings. He even rented an apartment above that of Mobile's "Imperial Wizard," Elmo Bernard, for surveillance purposes.

In the 1950s Mobile's Klan chapter openly promoted its race-baiting agenda. In the 1957 election for Imperial Wizard, Elmo Bernard, ran against Joseph Langan for City Commissioner. The campaign included a flier entitled "WHITE SUPREMACY NOW AND FOREVER." Bernard's campaign buttons depicted two Black men hanging from a tree, celebrating what was widely regarded as the most abhorrent event in Mobile's history.[26] Barnard lost but got 2,000 votes. In a city that prided itself on its racial tolerance, only Foley was taking on the Klan directly.

In 1954, under the leadership of Spring Hill president Andrew Smith, the college quietly challenged the Klan as well, enrolling nine Black students and becoming the first college in the Deep South to desegregate. It escaped any public attention but would remain the only one for another decade. Two years later, despite the Alabama backlash to the *Brown* decision requiring the desegregation of public schools, Autherine Lucy, with the legal help of the NAACP's Thurgood Marshall and a court order, entered the University of Alabama at Tuscaloosa. She was the first Black student to be admitted to a white public school or university in Alabama. She attended her first day of classes on Friday, February 3, 1956. The following Monday, more than one thousand rioters pelted the car that escorted her between classes, stoned the president's home, and made threats on her life. The university suspended her out of concern for her safety, and Marshall did not overturn that decision in the courts.

The backlash to the *Brown* decision propelled an upsurge in Klan activity in Mobile that had not been utilized in the Klan's Reconstruction Era–life. At Spring Hill College, Foley enlisted his students in surveying local opinions about the Klan. Of the six hundred respondents, 86 percent felt federal intervention was needed. After these results were reported in 1956, things escalated. A cross was burned in town, and Klan members spied from trees outside campus to monitor Foley's movements. After a bomb was set off in the yard of a Black family, Foley responded by placing a full-page ad in the *Mobile Register* calling for the curbing of Klan intimidation. In January 1957, a dozen Klan cars drove on campus planning to burn a kerosene-soaked cross outside one of the dormitories. Students, studying late for finals, appeared from the dorm and chased the Klan away before the cross could be lighted. The Klan retaliated, burning a cross at the front gate to the college. Commenting on the incident, President Smith struck a more measured tone than Foley, saying that he hoped "that a closer study of the divine meaning of the symbol which they sought to defame by burning would cause some to change their ways and cease to promote hatred and terror among people supposed to live in peace and harmony together bought for by the One who died on the Cross."[27]

Foley continued to seek racial justice through his actions and teaching until his death in 1990. He influenced many former students who went on to pursue similar goals. Martin Luther King, in his April 16, 1963, "Letter from a Birmingham Jail," singled out as an exception to the religious leaders of the state who warned against his "unwise and untimely" activities, "the Catholic leaders of Alabama for integrating Spring Hill College several years ago."[28]

Joseph Langan (1912–2004) broke the mold. Repeatedly elected in the Deep South, he was the only white local political official committed to racial justice. Langan's grandfather had joined the Irish exodus during the potato famines of the 1850s and ended up settling near where his grandson would help build the Mobile Civic Center.[29] As Joseph Langan explained it, poor Irish immigrants had little say and politics was a way to gain power: "Unless you had a voice in the community you didn't have anything. A lot of Irish began to organize, become voters and participate."[30] Langan started working in a grocery store to help support the family in fourth grade, going on to graduate from Murphy High in 1931 and then, eventually from Spring Hill College in 1951 where he would later serve as a board member.

His experiences in the Army during World War II, however, did the most to change him. He indignantly recalled a friend who had shared a trench with him but could not go into a restaurant with Langan on his return. Langan saw a Mobile bus pick up a white passenger at one corner and bypass a Black rider at the next. Enraged, he sent an indignant letter to the director of the transit system, telling him he thought he had gotten on the wrong boat coming back from overseas and ended up in Germany. After the war, he concluded, "you had to take sides." He did, becoming an ally of both LeFlore and Foley, involved in all the same legal suits about voter registration, city governance, transit, and school desegregation.

Through a coalition of Black and white liberals, Langan's ability to maintain office ended in 1969, as impatience with the slow pace of change and distrust grew. He left politics with a long list of civic accomplishments in a city with much-expanded boundaries. In 2009, six years after his death, the city dedicated Unity Point Park, a space on the historic boundary line between the white and Black sections of town that now features a large bronze statue of Langan and LeFlore standing together shaking hands.

Mobile and its racial politics are, however, too complicated to be represented by such a statue. Noble Beasley (1932–2014) never defined it that way. He and the organization he led, Neighborhood Organized Workers of Mobile (NOW), drew support from an impatient younger contingent of activists and undermined some of what

LeFlore and Langan thought they were accomplishing. LeFlore and Langan and Mobile's existing political establishment viewed Beasley as a dangerous, possibly criminal demagogue. NOW supporters portrayed him as a respected leader of Mobile's Black community. Married with children, his wife was a schoolteacher. Noble had worked for the post office, served as a merchant seaman, and also served in the Army. He owned and operated a popular night spot in town, the Sabre Club, which provided him with a degree of economic independence.[31] NOW's board included postal workers, teachers, and businessowners in Mobile. Leaders in Mobile had prided themselves on avoiding the national headlines about violent racial confrontations that were stigmatizing other Southern cities. NOW's conclusion was that a group of more conservative Black preachers, organized and carefully cultivated by the "White establishment," had told Martin Luther King not to come to Mobile, shifting attention elsewhere.[32] NOW went ahead to organize the first mass protest demonstration in Mobile's civil rights history only after Martin Luther King's assassination in 1968. The city denied the group a permit, but NOW marched anyway with a crowd of nine thousand mostly younger Black and white participants joining them. NOW also targeted the America's Junior Miss Pageant, a nationally televised event, with a protest that would lead to three hundred demonstrators being arrested. NOW even picketed Mardi Gras, the most sacred of Mobile's sacred cows, angering many.

In 1969, NOW organized a bitter challenge to Mobile's existing civil rights leadership—a boycott of the municipal election. Beasley argued that Langan and LeFlore were in the pocket of Mobile's white elite. The Pink Sheets that LeFlore used to endorse candidates supportive of Black community aspirations never guaranteed orally or in writing what white politicians would do for the Black community if elected. Individual voters, not LeFlore, should have the power to make that decision. The resulting low turnout proved fatal for the old coalition. It undermined LeFlore's ability to bolster Black influence in the election through his Pink Sheets, and they ceased to be distributed. Langan lost reelection as commissioner and never stood for election again. NOW would disappear within two years, leaving little to fill the void.

Noble Beasley, either through white establishment retaliation or his own actions, destroyed NOW. He had not just antagonized the conservative white establishment but also Langan, LeFlore, and other civil rights leaders who could have helped with his defense. He was first arrested on murder charges that later proved unfounded. Beasley was eventually convicted for life on charges that he "conspired" to sell a large amount of crack cocaine. As documented in an interview conducted after his release, the charges were never substantiated.[33] Nothing had come of the FBI surveillance of his activities, and the key incriminating witness at the trial was a "flipped" drug dealer who got a suspended sentence for his testimony. Beasley was convicted and spent forty years in federal prison, emerging only a year before his death from a heart attack at age eighty-two in 2014. (A bill, supported by President Biden, was introduced in 2021 to the US Congress. It would end the disparities in sentencing for crack and powder cocaine that, regardless of Beasley's guilt or innocence, contributed to the length of his sentence and, more broadly, to the overall racial disparities in incarceration rates. The bill failed to pass but its supporters still await a more opportune time for resubmission.) Remarkably, the taped interview after his release reveals how upbeat Beasley felt about what "they"—Mobile's Jim Crow challengers Langan, LeFlore, and Beasley—had been able to achieve "together."

Beasley's lengthy sentence and NOW's destruction, at least from the distance of time, just seems too connected to other questionable events beginning during this same period. It was the beginning of Nixon's "war on drugs" that proved interminable under later presidencies and produced a more than four-fold increase in male

incarceration rates and an even higher increase for Black and Hispanic people. A bitter quote from now-deceased John Ehrlichman,
who served as Nixon's White House Counsel and then Chief Domestic Advisor continues to resurface, originally obtained by journal-
ist Dan Baum. Most surviving NOW sympathizers shared a similar
assessment.

> "You want to know what this was really all about?" he asked with the
> bluntness of a man who, after public disgrace and a stretch in fed-
> eral prison, had little left to protect. "The Nixon campaign in 1968,
> and the Nixon White House after that, had two enemies: the anti-
> war left and black people. You understand what I'm saying? We knew
> we couldn't make it illegal to be either against the war or black, but
> by getting the public to associate the hippies with marijuana and
> blacks with heroin, and then criminalizing both heavily, we could
> disrupt those communities. We could arrest their leaders, raid their
> homes, break up their meetings, and vilify them night after night on
> the evening news. Did we know we were lying about the drugs? Of
> course we did.[34]

Were civil rights activists being punished by their adversaries who
could count on help from Nixon's war on drugs, Hoover's COIN-
TELPRO illegal campaign against "radical" groups, and prosecutors
just concerned about winning convictions to finish the job? Sonnie
Wellington Hereford, the Black physician and civil rights leader who
helped desegregate Huntsville Alabama, faced similar destruction
on drug related charges involving his prescription of pain killers for
Medicaid patients. Hereford's failure to exercise sufficient caution
in prescribing pain killers for his patients resulted in the permanent
revocation of his license by the Alabama Medical Review Board and
left him destitute.[35] In both cases, the harshness of the punishment
did not appear to fit the crime.

All four of these challengers to Jim Crow in Mobile faced the un-relenting persistence, skill, political connections, and ruthlessness of four defenders. These individuals milked the lost cause myths and never conceded. These opponents of civil rights included a novelist, a judge, a Klan leader, and a governor. In different ways, each figure illustrates why progress in ending Jim Crow was so torturous.

Augusta Evans Wilson (1835–1909) was a prominent proponent of the Confederate cause in Mobile. Her family had owned enslaved people, part of the "property" lost at the Civil War's end. She iden-tified with the Alabama owners of enslaved people and a nostalgic view of the antebellum era. As one of the most popular novelists of the nineteenth century, she served as an influential legitimizer of the "lost cause." Augusta would publish nine novels in her lifetime in the genre of "domestic or sentimental fiction" (traditionally coded as fe-male writers writing for female audiences). While critics found her books melodramatic and pretentious, she attracted a huge national following and most of her books became bestsellers. Her literary fame made her a prominent citizen and influential voice in Mobile where she lived most of her life.

She supported Alabama's secession from the Union in the Civil War and announced she was "ready to drain [her] veins rather than yield to the ignominious rule of black Republicanism."[36] Her actions matched her words. She served as a volunteer nurse and organized women volunteers to sew sandbags for Mobile's defenses. She also served as an advisor to influential Confederate politicians and gen-erals. That advice, unusual for a woman at that time, was not just about public relations matters but about military strategy as well, in-cluding the construction of Mobile defenses and the hiring and firing of generals. At the end of the war, she sheltered a Confederate Gen-eral in her home who was trying to escape capture by Union forces. After the war, Evans Wilson fundraised for the return of Mobile's Confederate dead to graves in their home city and for the erection of a monument to commemorate their sacrifice. She continued to oppose suffrage for Black men and all women for the rest of her life.

Her final fund-raising campaign in Mobile involved the establishment of a white-only hospital, the Mobile Infirmary. The hospital, constructed after her death, became the key defender against a federal offensive aimed at racially desegregating medical facilities in 1966. One imagines some of her spirit living on in that hospital's struggle. As acknowledged on the hospital's website, "Wilson led a series of fund-raising events from pencil sales, to craft bazaars and sewing circles—along with a $50,000 bond issue to fund the construction."[37] Her vision of a "charitable" white-only facility to serve primarily the upper class Mobile helped account for its growth in size and relative affluence. The hospital board and administrators' unwillingness to pressure its medical staff to desegregate in 1966 would play a central role in the death of Dr. Jean Cowsert.

No one, however, was more devoted to Alabama's white supremacist past and more effective in blocking an end to Jim Crow than Walter Burgwyn Jones (1888–1963), a member of one of the most prominent families in Alabama. His father, Thomas Goode Jones, achieved the rank of major in the Confederate Army and had the honor of delivering the flag of surrender from Lee to Grant at the end of the war. He would go on to serve as Speaker of the Alabama house of representatives and as governor, and serve as a representative to the constitutional convention that wrote Alabama's 1901 Constitution. Walter, at age fourteen, would join him at that convention as an observer and would later lavish praise on the participants' preservation of white supremacy.[38]

Walter Jones received a law degree from the University of Alabama. He was picked to serve as a judge of the Alabama Circuit Court in Montgomery in 1920. He would continue to serve in this capacity and later as presiding judge of the circuit until his death in 1963. He was an "institution" in Montgomery, as well known as the state capital and Jefferson Davis's home. He also served as editor of the *Alabama Lawyer*, from its start in 1940 until his death. A publication sponsored by the Alabama Bar Association, Jones freely used it to support white supremacy. His diatribes were influential in shaping the language and thinking of the legal community of Alabama.

After the 1954 *Brown v. Board of Education* Supreme Court decision, his court became a main stage in efforts to block civil rights challengers. In 1956, he granted an injunction against NAACP operations in the state of Alabama. The injunction, prepared secretly by state attorney general John Patterson in collaboration with Jones, demanded that the NAACP cease operations in Alabama or turn over a list of all its members. It claimed that the organization had harmed the citizens of Alabama by, among other things, supporting the Montgomery bus boycott and the admission of Autherine Lucy to the University of Alabama. The negative national publicity from these events, Patterson argued, had damaged the state's reputation. These activities, he also argued, were illegal because, although the NAACP had been working in the state since 1918, it was an "out of state business" that had failed to give the necessary information to the state to allow its operation. Jones imposed a fine of $10,000 that would be remitted if the NAACP supplied its membership list in five days or raise the fine to $100,000 if it did not. The NAACP gave most of the information demanded but it refused to supply its membership list. It feared retaliation against its members, as Patterson and Jones had every reason to expect it would. Checkmate—the NAACP had no choice but to cease operations in Alabama. The issues were litigated over the next eight years, including four hearings before the US Supreme Court that finally, expecting further obstruction, ruled directly in the NAACP's favor rather than remanding it back to the state courts.

Not one to shrink from what he regarded as a sacred battle, Jones found a way in his court to even threaten the survival of the *New York*

Times.[39] On March 29, 1960, a full-page ad appeared in the *Times* with the headline "HEED THEIR RISING VOICES," echoing the words of a *Times* editorial. Identified as "The Committee to Defend Martin Luther King and the Struggle for Freedom in the South" and including the names of all the VIPs supporting the civil rights movement, it asked for contributions. Several factual errors appeared in the ad for which the *Times* later published corrections and apologized personally. Three million dollars in libel suits against the *Times* by city and state officials followed, arguing that their reputations had been damaged by this false information.[40] The suits, which some believed had been planned in the judge's chamber, were crafted to avoid federal authority and would be tried in Jones's circuit court.

A judge serving a less impartial role in such cases would be hard to find. The author of the *Confederate Creed*, Jones said, among other things, "I see in the Stars and Bars, the glorious banner of the Confederacy, as it waves in the Southern Breeze, a symbol of freedom and devotion to constitutional rights, an emblem of honor and character."[41] In 1961 the centennial of the Confederacy's founding was celebrated in Montgomery. Judge Jones swore in Jefferson Davis in the reenactment. Some of the jurors in a real trial in his court took part as well, and Jones seated them in the jury box in their Confederate reenactment uniforms. Seats in his courtroom were segregated.

The libel cases against the *Times*, first by the city commissioner of Montgomery, came dangerously close to serving their intended purpose. The total claims exceeded three million dollars and potentially threatened to intimidate the national press and broadcasters from covering the Southern civil rights protests. It took almost four years for the Supreme Court to reverse the Alabama courts' claims. The landmark decision added protection for the press against libel suits brought by public officials, which is essential in an open democracy (*New York Times Co. v. Sullivan* 376 (US) 254 [1964]). Judge Jones had died a year earlier, not living to experience this defeat, and joining his Confederate comrades from earlier battles. Sarah Palin lost in a similar unsuccessful libel trial against the *New York Times* in 2022.[42]

It is easy to portray Robert Shelton (1929–2003) as Mr. Hyde for the defensive side of white supremacy. He had none of the patrician background, deep involvement in religious and civic affairs, or professed commitment to the rule of law that Judge Jones and Augusta Evans Wilson claimed. He made a living as a factory worker at BF Goodrich, as a car-tire salesperson, and as an operator of a small printing business in Tuscaloosa. Within the Klan movement, however, he proved an exceptionally skillful organizer, riding the tide of infighting to become the leader of its largest splinter group.[43] Morris Dees, one of the founders of the Southern Poverty Law Center, in Montgomery, once described Shelton as "America's most dangerous neo-Nazi."[44]

After being ousted from the US Klan in 1960, Shelton quickly drew chapters away from it to his new organization, the Alabama Knights of the Ku Klux Klan. That organization merged the following year into the United Klan of America with Shelton leading as the Imperial Wizard. At its height in the mid 1960s, his organization had about thirty thousand dues-paying members and as many as 250,000 more informal supporters.

The organization under Shelton's leadership was connected to most of the more notorious incidents of violence intended to intimidate, harass, and even murder Black and white supporters of civil rights efforts in the 1960s in Alabama.[45] These included interfering with the interstate travel of Freedom Riders in 1961 by setting ablaze their Greyhound bus and then beating them in the Birmingham and Montgomery bus stations; dynamiting the Sixteenth Street Baptist Church in Birmingham, killing four Black children; randomly killing a Black man, US Army Reservist Colonel Lemuel Penn, traveling on an interstate highway in Georgia in 1964; shooting and killing a white woman, Viola Liuzzo, who was transporting a Black civil rights worker on an interstate highway in Alabama in 1965; shooting into the Childersburg, Alabama, home of local NAACP chapter president Charles Woods in 1979 by thirteen members; flogging a Black man, Leon Richard Jarrett, in 1979 by thirteen members; and running Danny Adams off a state highway and beating him for his interracial marriage in 1980 by a financial supporter of the United Klan, Jimmy Dan Kilgore. Some of the participants in each of these crimes had been tried and found guilty. Some of the crimes could not have taken place without Shelton's consent. The promotional materials produced and distributed by his headquarters graphically supported such acts of violence.

Yet until the events of the night of March 20, 1981, in Mobile, Alabama, the United Klan of America and its leader Grand Wizard Robert Shelton had eluded responsibility for any of this racial terror. The lynching of nineteen-year-old Michael Donald in March 1981 by several members of the local Klavern, a unit of organization akin to a lodge used by the Klan, changed this. Donald was picked out randomly to serve as a warning for the acquittal of a Black man accused of the murder of a police officer. Donald's murder staggered the city. That the last recorded racial lynching in Alabama would take place in Mobile seemed inconceivable. Two local Klan members were tried and convicted by an all-white jury. One received a death sentence. But Shelton and his United Klan of America were left untouched.

A civil action in federal district court followed against Shelton and the United Klan of America. The local Mobile branch of the NAACP and the Alabama State Conference of NAACP branches joined Donald's mother, Mrs. Beulah Mae Donald, as plaintiffs. Morris Dees and the Southern Poverty Law Center served as their legal representatives. Their presentation to an all-white jury used all the connections between Shelton and the United Klan of America's misdeeds. The prosecution made good use of the graphic material included in the *Fiery Cross* newsletter encouraging such lynchings, which Shelton had produced as editor and publisher. For the jury, the graphic images of lynching proved devastating for Shelton.[46] The jury returned in a little more than four hours, awarding Ms. Donald seven million dollars.

The verdict bankrupted the United Klan of America and precipitated Shelton's resignation as its leader. In 1994 Shelton told an Associated Press reporter, "The Klan is my belief, my religion. But it won't work anymore. The Klan is gone forever."[47] Ms. Donald was able to retrieve only a small fraction of the amount awarded by the court from the liquidated assets of the Klan and died soon afterward. A reclusive and secretive Klan leader, Shelton completed the rest of his life in obscurity dying of a heart attack at age seventy-three in 2003. His daughter was embarrassed by his role in civil rights violence, and his son insisted that his own views were "totally opposite" but downplayed the negative aspects of the Klan. "To me," the son said, "he was always just a father and that's all he will ever be."[48] The hate and white supremacy ideology that fueled the growth of the United Klan of America, unfortunately, lives on in new iterations.

George Wallace (1919–1998) certainly leads the list of Alabama defenders of Jim Crow. A scrappy, scrawny five-foot-seven at Barbour County High School, he served as its football team's quarterback and won two state bantam weight Golden Glove titles. His addiction to the adrenaline rush of athletic combat was soon transferred to the thrill of political battles. He knew how to use all the stored up resentments of Reconstruction and the Great Depression to achieve overwhelming political victories.[49] He loomed over the civil rights era, serving a record-breaking four terms as governor, and he still elicits strong memories from former supporters and opponents. In his first inauguration speech as governor in 1963 he stood in the same spot that Jefferson Davis had stood when he was sworn in as president of the Confederacy and uttered the often repeated words (attributed to his speech writer, Ku Klux Klan leader and author of best seller fiction, Asa Earl Carter): "In the name of the greatest people who have ever trod the earth, I draw a line in the dust and toss the gauntlet before the feet of tyranny and I say segregation now, segregation tomorrow and segregation forever." He also "stood in the doorway," symbolically blocking the enrollment of two Black students at the University of Alabama in Tuscaloosa, and in 1965 he engaged in tense negotiations with LBJ concerning the Selma-to-Montgomery march for voting rights.

Wallace's success in a third-party presidential run in 1968 changed national politics. He captured the electoral votes of five Southern states and eroded the Democratic party's white, blue-collar support in the North. It probably did more to stall progress in ending Jim Crow than any other event. Later successful Republican presidential candidates Richard Nixon, Ronald Reagan, George H. W. Bush, George W. Bush, and Donald Trump benefitted from using Wallace's style and messages, albeit with the racism more coded.

In the late 1970s Wallace announced that he was a born-again Christian and apologized for his past segregationist stands. In an unannounced visit in 1979 to the Dexter Avenue Church in Montgomery—the church where King had served as pastor and organized the bus boycott —he told the congregation, "I have learned what suffering means. I think I can understand some of the pain Black people have come to endure. I know I contributed to it and can only ask forgiveness."[50] Of the four defenders of Jim Crow described here, he was the only one to apologize. Wallace had done more to perpetuate Jim Crow than Robert Shelton, who at least had to pay for some of the damage. Wallace had one more campaign for governor in 1982 and now wanted the Black vote. He got it and it contributed to his victory. Joseph Langdon, former Mobile commissioner and mayor, a bitter opponent of Wallace, believed that this conversion was no surprise. Wallace was just a politician counting votes and now the

Black votes counted. Did that make any final assessment of him better or worse?

Wallace's own children struggled with that question. His daughter Peggy published a wrenching memoir. She came to believe deeply in the cause of racial justice and her father's conversion to it. She marched hand in hand with Congressman John Lewis over the Edmund Petrus bridge in Selma in commemoration of the original Selma march. Peggy spoke in 2017 to the Congressional delegation at the Alabama Archives in Montgomery. The moderator asked John Lewis to say a few words about his impression of George Wallace. Congressman Lewis looked directly at Peggy, paused and said, "How could I possibly say anything bad about George Wallace, when this is his daughter?"[51] She was, as far as he was concerned, Wallace's most important legacy.

Wallace left mixed legacies for Mobile. On the one hand, he helped create the University of Southern Alabama, improving access to first-generation college students both Black and white. On the other, a tunnel named in his honor under the Bay accelerated white flight from Mobile's public schools. Wallace, at least in his public acts, tops the list of defenders of Jim Crow and belongs in the company of Augusta Evans Wilson, Walter B. Jones, and Robert Shelton. Their legacy persists.

The Mobile Jean Cowsert Faced on Her Return

Jean Cowsert returned to Mobile in 1959, when not an inch had been conceded in the war over Jim Crow. The 1901 constitutional restrictions on Black enfranchisement were still in place. The most explosive desegregation issue, school desegregation, had yet to be even raised. Masterfully designed, the Constitution never mentions race as a requirement that would have invited federal intrusion. Both the battles over disenfranchisement and desegregating public schools in Mobile dragged on long after Jean Cowsert's return, never to be fully resolved. Progress has always been fragile. Enfranchisement and school desegregation in Mobile illustrate difficulties not that different than what one would expect in health care.

The voting eligibility rules in that 1901 Constitution had their intended effect, and little had changed. In 1900, there were 183,000 Black voters registered in Alabama, but by 1903 that number had sunk to fewer than 3,000.[52] The voter suppression system prescribed in the 1901 Constitution continued to adapt, adding new obstacles. For example, registration times were limited to peak harvesting time to make it more difficult for tenant farmers in rural counties. The most effective measures, however, were the unwritten ones involving demeaning treatment and intimidation. In Mobile, a half century after the enactment of the 1901 Constitution, Black citizens still had to enter through the back "Colored" entrance of the Registration Office building, stand while white applicants had seats, and wait while all the white applicants were served first. Treatment got worse after the local NAACP chapter began to challenge such practices. In 1944 Napoleon Rivers, an elderly NAACP board member, after waiting and then demanding to speak to the chairman of the Board of Registrars, was dragged out of the building by the police officer on duty and thrown down the steps, fracturing his jaw and skull. The policeman then picked him up and arrested him for disorderly conduct.[53]

Even when successful in overcoming registration hurdles, Black citizens were still blocked from voting in the primaries until 1944. Alabama's Democratic party dominated state politics and excluded Black people from membership. The only votes that mattered were cast in white-only primaries. As if it were an elite private club, not a public part of the electoral process, party leaders insisted that they were free to choose their own members.

The only enfranchisement breakthrough had come in 1944 when

the Supreme Court put an end to Southern white primaries. Lonnie Smith, a Black dentist from Houston, sued a county election official, S. S. Allwright, over the Texas white primary, arguing that his constitutional rights under the Fourteenth and Fifteenth Amendments were violated. In a watershed 9–1 decision. the Supreme Court ruled in favor of Smith (*Smith v. Allwright*, US 321 649 [1944]). NAACP lawyer Thurgood Marshall regarded it as his most important case.[54]

Marshall, expecting Alabama's reaction, asked local NAACP chapters to assess the implementation of the *Smith* decision. LeFlore and other members of the Mobile NAACP brought along a *Life* magazine photographer as they tried to vote in the Democratic primary. Arms folded, a deputy sheriff blocked their entrance. "Haven't you heard of the Supreme Court ruling?" LeFlore asked. "This is Alabama, whites only," the deputy sheriff replied. The photo and story ran in *Life* the next week.[55] Lawsuits followed.

Members of Alabama's Democratic Party' understood that they would just have to find a way to blunt the Smith decision's impact on Black voting eligibility. Senator Boswell introduced what became the "Boswell Amendment." Voter applicants had to be able to correctly interpret a section of the US Constitution. County election registrars made these determinations, but no one tried to hide their intent. Boswell, who introduced the amendment in the State Senate, made that clear: "I feel if it is adopted Alabama will be assured white supremacy for another fifty years at least, the Supreme Court of the United States, to the contrary notwithstanding."[56] Former State Senator J. Thomas Heflin, one of the framers of the 1901 Constitution, was blunter: "The Boswell Amendment will keep scores of ignorant vicious Negro votes from being cast. No white man will be embarrassed by its adoption. It is purely and wholly in the interest of white supremacy."[57]

The more liberal wing of the party, including then state senator Joseph Langan opposed the Boswell Amendment as a fruitless embarrassment. The more dominant conservative wing, however, launched a campaign that included an ad in *Alabama* magazine pleading to "Help save our Alabama Black Belt from Negro Domination." It was promoted by the chairman of the State Democratic Executive committee as a "way to fight for white supremacy in our state and to make the Democratic Party of Alabama the White Man's Party."[58] While the Boswell Amendment lost decisively in Mobile, it won with 54 percent of the vote statewide.

The vote on the amendment had its intended effect. Three months afterward, the *Mobile Register* published a story indicating that since its passage almost all Black applicants for voter registration in Mobile had been rejected.[59] In the first two years after its implementation 2,800 white residents in Mobile County were registered, but only 104 Black voters, despite the concerted efforts of local civil rights groups. About 36 percent of the county's population was Black in 1946, but they represented only 2 percent of the registered voters.[60]

On January 7, 1949, the US District Court ruled that the "Boswell Amendment" was unconstitutional. A new version, dubbed "Boswell Jr.," was proposed, which replaced the implausible constitutional "understanding" clause with one that required potential voters to "be of good character and embrace the duties and obligations of citizenship under the constitution of the United States." This new ruse was defeated by a filibuster by then state senator Joseph Langan. In 1951, however, the state legislature adopted a "new" voter qualification law that required potential voters to be able to read or write any section of the Constitution, be of good character, and swear that they were not part of any group or agency devoted to overthrowing the government. It also tried to conceal the capriciousness of local registrar decisions by requiring the state supreme court to produce a standardized questionnaire that local registrars should use in making their eligibility determinations. That law stood on the books along with all the other forms of informal intimidation by white local registrars until the passage of the Voting Rights Act of 1965. Enacted just a week after Medicare, the Selma to Montgomery March spurred its passage. It prohibited all the state-enforced practices that had a disproportionate impact on Black voter registration. It imposed federal oversight of the voter registration process on Alabama and five other states with histories of Black voter suppression. Sadly, these enfranchisement struggles continue.[61]

Mobile also supplies a useful case study to highlight the difficulties of school desegregation. A county-wide district, the largest in Alabama, Mobile included almost a cross-section of the United States—an urban core, suburban and rural areas—and a total of 1,644 square miles. Mobile was the focus of the longest and most bitter civil rights class action lawsuit over school segregation in the country. *Birdie Mae Davis et al. v. Board of School Commissioners of Mobile County* began in 1963, just while Cowsert was hitting a stride in her practice in Mobile. It ended in 1997, thirty years after her death. As elsewhere, its aspirational roots were in the 1954 *Brown v. Board of Education* decision and its accomplishments in the light of that decision disappointing.

Local civil rights activists understood how difficult implementing the *Brown* decision would be in Mobile and focused on easier targets, such as public accommodations. The *Brown* decision in Alabama produced immediate, determined, and skillful resistance. A state law passed in 1955 gave absolute authority to the local school board in student assignment to schools. Concerns about avoiding "social disruption" were included as one of the criteria boards could use in making such decisions but race, of course, was not mentioned. A state constitutional amendment followed in 1956 allowing the school board to sell its schools to private entities if that was the only choice left to prevent racial integration.

The first challenge to school segregation in Mobile came in 1956 from Dorothy Danner, who had no idea what she was getting herself into. She came from a wealthy Mobile family, far more oblivious to all the obstacles of desegregation than Cowsert could have possibly been.[62] Born in Mobile, the only daughter of a family in the timber processing industry, her mother died when she was fourteen. Characterized by relatives as "difficult," she completed college at Vassar, graduating in 1939 and then moved to Greenwich Village. She returned to Mobile and her father's home toward the end of World War II. She would make poor choices in three marriages and dabble in civil rights, pacifism, and animal rights causes. Her first husband, a Dutch national and heavy drinker, killed himself just six months after the wedding with the gun given to him by her father as a Christmas present. Shortly afterward, she became interested in helping the six-year-old daughter of the household maid, Carrie Mae McCants. She took the child as her ward to Europe for several years and Carrie attended several of the finer private schools there. Carrie Mae would return to Mobile in time to enter eighth grade in the fall of 1956. Used to having her way as a member of Mobile's privileged royalty, Danner sent a note to the president of the Mobile County School Board requesting Carrie Mae's admission to a white school. The request was brusquely refused. After the story of her application appeared in the local paper, a caravan of cars with about one hundred robed Klansman arrived at the driveway of her home with horns blaring.[63] They erected and burned a ten-foot cross. Obscene phone calls, threats, and another cross burning at the house of a friend followed. A salacious rumor circulated that the young girl was really Danner's daughter and her husband's discovery of this illicit interracial affair precipitated his suicide, and this further ostracized Danner. School integration was not going to be an easy path to follow for those interested in more than just tilting at windmills.

In November 1962, John LeFlore and the parents of some Black students petitioned to enter Mobile's white schools and began a more serious effort. In March 1963, nine years after the *Brown* decision, the Nonpartisan Voters League, standing for the parents of twenty-three children in the county's school system filed a class action lawsuit in federal district court, *Birdie Mae Davis et al. v. Board of School Commissioners of Mobile County.* LeFlore argued that the County was running an illegal dual school system and looked to end the assignment of students to schools by race. It was the first legal challenge to public school segregation in Alabama, and the League was taking on the largest school district in the state.[64]

Federal District Court judge Daniel Davis presided over the case for its first eight years. He was an appointee of President Truman and sympathetic to the desegregation cause. The Mobile County School Board was determined to block any efforts to end segregation. "Over the years," the superintendent assured them, "it has been the purpose of all of our staff to give the Board every possible support in achieving the objective of maintaining segregated schools."[65] The school district's response to desegregation demands began in the fall of 1963. Token desegregation of the white schools was combined with "freedom of choice." There would be no forced assignment to assure desegregation. "Freedom of choice" meant preservation of segregation since no one would do anything they didn't want to do, and intimidation would influence those "choices." The plan's implementation began in the fall of 1963 with two Black seniors attending Murphy High School, Mobile's white high school. (Murphy had been the high school alma mater of Dorothy Danner, Joseph Langan, and Jean Cowsert). The plan was to go ahead with the token desegregation of one lower grade each year. The fears of white parents were minimized and it responded, if only minimally, to the plaintiff demands.

The plan did not, however, prevent Governor George Wallace from "drawing another line in the sand," issuing an executive order preventing the two students from enrolling, and sending state troopers to block them. President Kennedy countered by federalizing the

Alabama state guard and a federal court order forbidding the governor from interfering. Despite the governor's intervention, this token step integrating the two Black students went ahead but the issue of "true" integration would linger on.

The civil rights struggle in Mobile, just as elsewhere, was defined as a no holds barred "us versus them" battle. It ceased to have anything to do with working out an accommodation in everyone's self-interest. Alabama's ratification of the 1901 Constitution involved most poor white residents voting for their own disenfranchisement. Appeals to racial animus blinded most poor voters from acting in their own self-interest.[66]

In *The Sum of Us*, Heather McGhee provides devastating examples in the fate of public swimming pools in southern communities during the 1950s and '60s.[67] A source of civic pride, public swimming pools had expanded across the South as gathering places and respite from summer heat into the 1950s. The Oak Park pool in Montgomery, Alabama, was the crown jewel of the Parks Department and the finest one in the area. In 1959, however, the federal courts ruled that Montgomery's segregated parks and their pools were unconstitutional. Just as in so many instances elsewhere, the city council chose to close the pool rather than integrate it. The parks were closed, the pools drained and filled in. Even after the city parks opened again on an integrated basis a decade later, the Oak Park pool was never rebuilt. Who won and who lost? Black access did not win, but most white residents in Montgomery did not either. They could not afford to build their own pool or join one of the town's private country clubs, so they lost out too.

The same ill logic played out in Macon, Georgia as well. A hand from the grave destroyed a beautiful, much-loved community park.[68] US senator Augustus Bacon, who died in 1914, left sixty acres in his will to Macon as a "park and pleasure ground" to be used by "white women, white girls, white boys and white children." Bacon's Field, as the park was named, was a heavily wooded sixty-acre track soon transformed with trails and known for its lush magnolias. The city's parks department added a swimming pool, tennis courts, a petting zoo for children, and a clubhouse used by women's groups in the city for meetings. The federal Works Progress Administration (WPA) in the 1930s supplied the labor for some of this development. A 1963 federal court decision ordered the end to segregated public parks. The predictable resistance by Macon city officials followed: the pool was closed, the animals in the petting zoo shipped elsewhere, and the city tried to transfer the park to private hands. A Supreme Court decision in 1965 ruled that the city could not get off the hook; it was still a public park and would have to be used on an unsegregated basis. However, there was the matter of the "intent" in Bacon's will. Bacon could not have predicted the later court ruling. Bacon's heirs insisted that a racially integrated park violated the will's intent, and the land had to be returned to them for sale. The attorney general of Georgia supported leaving it as a city park for all Georgians, but the Supreme Court of Georgia ruled that Bacon wanted an all-white park or no park at all and the property was returned to the owner-ship of his heirs. It had been a public park for fifty years, developed with public funds. None of the distant heirs lived in the area any-more, but the decision resulted in an effortless windfall for them. The property was sold to developers, the area stripped, denuded of trees and shrubbery but with plenty of room for asphalt parking in what became the Baconfield Shopping Center. The Shopping Center did not fare well as a long-term business venture; some of the store-fronts are now empty and it has become a public eyesore.

On the brighter side, Mobile did succeed in integrating its pub-lic golf course rather than closing it. It was quickly desegregated in response to a federal court order in 1964. Perhaps Mobile golfers are more obsessed about their golf game than matters of race. An earlier battle over integrating the public golf course in Greensboro,

North Carolina, at about the same time did not progress as smoothly. George Simkins, DDS, the Greensboro dentist who would later bring the suit that would begin the drive to desegregate the nation's hospitals, first sued to desegregate Greensboro's golf course. Simkins won but, according to account some white residents in Greensboro were sore losers:

> Two days before integration was to take effect the club house mysteriously burned down. The fire marshal went out and condemned the whole golf course. It stayed condemned for seven years. Of course, that denied access to white golfers, so nobody could play and that made them mad too. Finally, after seven years it was opened on an integrated basis.[69]

Perhaps the fire marshal was not a golfer.

Closing public swimming pools and golf courses was just the beginning. Lack of public investment in childcare, education, and health insurance sets the United States apart from most developed nations in the world. More white citizens than Black suffer from that underinvestment, just as more were disenfranchised by the 1901 Alabama Constitution. No one won, including the wealthy elites, from such "public solidarity" investments. Perhaps medicine in Mobile could do better.

CHAPTER SIX

Jim Crow Medicine

THE TRAIN GROUND TO A HALT at the Plateau station in North Mobile in 1919. Known as Africatown, the last illegally transported enslaved persons from Africa landed near here just before the Civil War. They forged a freed community here after the War. James Franklin, MD, a thirty-three-year-old Black man, climbed off the train. He walked down the street carrying his doctor's bag.

Franklin had been practicing medicine in Evergreen, Alabama. It was 1919 and the influenza pandemic had taken its toll. The wife of a white farmer was sick. Desperate, and unable to get help from the white doctor in town, he pleaded with Franklin. Franklin helped and the farmer believed that the doctor saved her life. The Klan found out. A Black man touching a white woman's body could not be tolerated. A mob gathered to lynch him.[1] The farmer rushed him to the next train, paying his fare. Franklin escaped alive but penniless, with nothing but his doctor's bag.

He had always prevailed. Franklin escaped childhood poverty in Chattanooga, Tennessee, and worked his way through Lincoln University outside Philadelphia by waiting on tables. Graduating with a straight A average in 1911, Franklin entered the University of Michigan Medical School in Ann Arbor.[2] He would work his way through as did all but one of about thirty-nine Black students enrolled at the university at the time—waiting on tables, tutoring, and other odd jobs. The campus paper, the *Michigan Daily*, noted with pride, as a measure of Michigan's commitment to "democracy, brotherhood and equality," that the number of Black students enrolled at Michigan ranked third among historically white institutions in the country.[3] There was no on-campus housing, and students had to rent rooms in private homes that largely segregated them by race. Franklin gained membership in Alpha Phi Alpha, the Black fraternity. He lived in their fraternity house on Ingalls Street during his final year. Franklin graduated in 1914 near the top of his medical class. His need to work to cover the cost of his education limited his involvement in the usual extracurricular activities graduating students are credited with. He was the only Black student in a graduating medical class of thirty-seven. One woman graduated in his class.

Franklin served in World War I in a medical unit in the US Army in Kentucky, caring for Black recruits. He was, however, assigned the title "Sergeant" rather than "Doctor," an indignity he would resent for the rest of his life.

He soon had a thriving practice in Mobile with patients standing in line outside his office. Just as other Black doctors in the Jim Crow South, the demand for his services translated into a comfortable living and social status within Mobile's Black community. He continued to make house calls, accepted whatever payment or exchange a patient could supply, and never turned anyone away. Franklin soon moved his practice to Davis Avenue (later renamed Martin Luther King Jr. Avenue) in Mobile and bought a seven-bedroom home several blocks away. *Ebony Magazine* listed him in 1954 as "the South's richest Negro doctor." His accumulated real estate holdings would include two three-story office buildings, seventeen houses, and two pharmacies. The exclusion of Black customers from hotel accommodations in Mobile resulted in him hosting visiting Black celebrities in his home, including Marian Anderson, Paul Robeson, Thurgood Marshall, Jackie Robinson, Roy Campanella, and Walter White, president of the NAACP. Klan threats followed a stay by White because its members assumed his light complexion meant he was white.

None of Dr. Franklin's relative wealth, professional credentials, or social status made any difference in opening doors to the expanding resources available to the white medical profession in Mobile. The Mobile medical society excluded Black physicians, as did all the city's hospitals. His patients were largely shut out of this world as well. He might refer a patient to a white doctor who had hospital privileges but there were few beds allocated for Black patients and it was an uncertain one-way street. Franklin left the direct-action protest to his wife, Marguerite, who took part in Mobile lunch counter sit-ins, train station desegregation, and once managed to evade the Klan in a car chase. The medical Jim Crow caste system was just beginning to break down as Dr. Franklin made his will in 1972. "Now, I don't want you going through my books to collect any money from those that owe me," he told his wife. "When I'm dead, my bills are paid. People have paid me everything they need to pay me."[4] He died shortly afterward on the way to make a house call.

Denied hospital privileges to the end, he had earned a special place of honor in Mobile's Black community. His office was transformed into the first site of the Franklin Memorial Health Center in 1975. Franklin Memorial has since expanded to include twenty-six sites with more than 255 employees.[5] Federal funds supported the center and its expansion. The center was part of one of the more successful initiatives to grow out of President Lyndon Johnson's Office of Economic Opportunity. It was modeled after a similar program developed earlier in South Africa during the apartheid regime to overcome the lack of Black access to medical care. The federal Health Resources and Services Administration now funds about 1,400 such health centers operating 13,000 delivery sites serving thirty million patients.[6] An expansion of the program was included in the 2010 Affordable Care Act. What was conceived as a temporary "safety net" has proven to be an enduring necessity of the American health system with strong bipartisan support. The program supplies direct federal payments to the centers, circumventing state and municipal control and requiring governing boards whose majority representatives must be patients of the center. The Franklin Memorial Health Center honors its namesake, but one could ask whether it means we are still living in an apartheid world like the one that inspired this model of care.

Mobile's Medical Society

The Medical Society of Mobile County exerted a powerful grip on the development of health care in Mobile. Dr. Josiah Nott founded the society in 1841, the first of its kind in Alabama. He would go on to help create the state medical society and found Alabama's first medical school, the Alabama College of Medicine in Mobile in 1859. His contribution to the Mobile County Medical Society is still acknowledged on its website. Nott was a forceful spokesperson for white supremacy and the inferiority of other races. Black physicians were excluded from membership in the county and state medical societies he helped create. Organized like an exclusive private club, the medical society looked to assure tight-knit bonds among members. A few negative votes were enough to exclude a candidate from membership. According to Dr. Samuel Eichold, II, founder of Mobile's Medical Museum, the elections were conducted with the traditional "blackball" method used in similar fraternal groups at the time, with each member given a white or a black ball to cast into an urn. Several black balls were enough to reject the physician from membership.[7] The predictable effect was to both silence dissention and concentrate power among a few members with longer tenure.

Hospital medical staff in Mobile were "open" to all medical society members. Physicians on a hospital's staff might be disciplined for their failure to update medical records or share in the responsibilities for other hospital medical staff member duties. The ultimate certification of their medical competence, specialty privileges, and ethical integrity necessary for membership on any hospital medical staff in the city rested with the medical society.

The individual physician chose which hospital to send a patient to be admitted. That choice depended on the race, religion, and insurance status of the patient. The central location of the hospitals, convenient to doctors who had privileges at all of them, helped support this physician "freedom of choice." The fiction was that the "choice" of hospital was up to the patient, but that decision was usually made by his physician. Thus, not only did the medical society control the hospital privileging process but the admission process as well. The members of the medical society could preserve hospital segregation of patients just by exercising their "freedom of choice" of where they admitted patients without the hospital having any direct say in the matter. A hospital could remain segregated without ever discriminating by race. They just admitted the patients referred to them by members of their medical staff.

The whole statewide regulatory infrastructure, licensure of physicians, hospitals, and public health surveillance had its origins in the Medical Society of Mobile County. Jerome Cochran, "the Father of Alabama public health," began practice in Mobile in 1865, joining its medical society. He built an unusually close relationship between the society and the public health infrastructure in the state, helping to set up a state medical society and a state health department, a board of medical examiners, and a licensure commission. As state health officer he devoted most of his career to fighting outbreaks of yellow fever, smallpox, typhoid, diphtheria, and cholera. He gained a national reputation for fighting such epidemics through the laws of quarantine, anticipating the scientific findings by as much as twenty to forty years.

Each hospital faced heated medical staff conflicts. Hospitals were becoming increasingly important as physicians specialized. Who was allowed to do what made all the difference in how much income physicians could make. Challenges to the old guard medical society leadership over specialty credentialing came to a head with the return of medical veterans and recently trained specialists setting up practices in Mobile after World War II. The challenges involved conflicts over who was permitted to do particular procedures and how ethical abuses that were financially profitable could be eliminated. According to this new cohort, reflected in oral histories provided after their retirement, there was plenty of house cleaning to be done.[8] Some felt that these older leaders had used their authority to get rid of competition by selecting which physicians would be drafted and shipped off for military service so the mercenary inner circle could make more money. Many returning veterans found their reentry to civilian practice delayed by "blackballing" from certain medical society members.

General practitioners lacking formal training were doing surgery, grandfathered in with the blessings of the leadership of the Mobile County Medical Society. Arthur A. Wood, MD, Mobile native and Tulane-trained surgeon, returned from World War II only to confront a major political battle over the way surgical specialists were getting hospital surgical privileges. A small group of influential older physicians held sway. Most of the members of the credential committee making these decisions, all closely allied with the old guard leaders, had served in this capacity for more than twenty years, Wood ran for election to the credential committee and won narrowly. The first thing he did was demand a vote by the full membership to restrict service on the committee to not exceed two three-year terms. The motion was passed by the medical society and board control by the old guard was broken. More formalized credentialing requirements were imposed.

The newcomers to surgical practices in Mobile found rampant abuses. "Ghost surgery," turning the surgery over to assistants without privileges and without the consent of the patient was common. Many of the newcomers were reluctant participants. According to Ernest D. DeBakey, MD, who began his surgical practice in Mobile in 1948, "there was a lot of unnecessary surgery going on and we created a surgery committee at the Infirmary and Dr. Wert, the pathologist at the hospital spearheaded it and helped stop it. We put the hospital on a higher level."[9] For all the internal frictions, the Mobile Medical Society solved its own problems. Federal intrusion in the practice of medicine in Mobile would come over the issue of racial segregation and would face forceful, united medical society opposition.

Mobile's Hospitals

Mobile's hospitals grew as an extension of its medical society. They operated in a strict Jim Crow world. White medical society members served as a bridge allowing their Black patients to enter segregated parts of that hospital world. As in most urban areas in the United States, Mobile's five original hospitals reflected the history of three different evolving concerns shaping their creation: (1) controlling the problems posed by "others," (2) caring for "one's own," and (3) assuring equity. The first two hospitals, Mobile City Hospital and the US Marine Hospital, were public entities concerned with the poor and exercising community control over the spread of infectious diseases. The second two were voluntary charitable enterprises, Providence Hospital, and the Mobile Infirmary, concerned with serving the medical needs involved in "taking care of our own." The fifth and final facility, Blessed St. Martin de Porres, tried to address the needs of those that had been left out—Black physicians and their patients. Its creation, as similar facilities in other communities, ushered the beginning of the medical civil rights era in Mobile.

Mobile City Hospital (1831), just as those founded in other American cities, focused on caring for the indigent who could not be cared for in their own homes. They functioned as poor and pest houses. Most people suffering from illnesses were treated at home by family members but smallpox, yellow fever, and malaria wreaked havoc with such arrangements.

Mobile City Hospital operations were also shaped by the Sisters of Charity, which managed it under contract. Nott and other Mobile County Medical Society leaders further shaped the development of Mobile City by getting court approval to set up the Mobile School of Medicine in 1859. Funds for the construction of a four-story building to house it followed from the state legislature in 1860. Mobile City Hospital would serve its faculty as a teaching site until the decision was made to move the medical school to the University of Alabama in 1920.

Mobile would regain a medical school and shift the ownership of Mobile City Hospital (later renamed University Hospital) with the creation of the University of Southern Alabama medical school in 1970. The facility became the first structure acquired in what would become an expanding medical complex.

Mobile's US Marine Hospital (1842) would join the Maritime Hospital System. It was established by an Act of Congress in 1798, as both the nation's first attempt at supplying a defense against infectious diseases and a way to pay for patient care. A tax on seaman's wages helped finance the network of hospitals along the nation's coastal shipping arteries. The hospitals mostly served as guard houses protecting against the spread of infectious diseases. Mobile's facility also served briefly in military crises, caring for Union and Confederate casualties during the Civil War and US military ones during World War I. With the growth of vaccines, antibiotics, and international air travel the Marine Hospital in Mobile outlived its original purpose. One of Mobile's most imposing nineteenth century structures, it was repurposed after being decommissioned and now serves as the Mobile County Health Department headquarters. Part of it was refurbished in 1984 as the Major General William C. Gogas Clinic, in honor of the Mobile native and physician who battled to eradicate yellow fever and malaria in occupied Havana and in the construction of the Panama Canal. The entire national network of infectious disease Marine hospitals closed or were repurposed a half century ago.

Providence Hospital (1855) was set up because of the activities of the Sisters of Charity in Mobile. Elizabeth Ann Seton, later named the first American born saint of the Catholic Church, founded the Sisters of Charity of St. Joseph, in Emmitsburg, Maryland in 1809. Part of an order dedicated to serving the poor, it was asked by the first bishop of Mobile, Michael Portier, to help care for the children orphaned by Mobile's yellow fever epidemic in 1841. Four sisters traveled to Mobile and the orphan asylum, known as St. Mary's Home, was set up shortly afterward. The sisters were soon asked to manage the city's hospital, but anti-Catholic sentiments briefly ended that arrangement in 1852. In the interim, local Catholic leaders pressed the sisters to open their own facility for Mobile's Catholic community. That two-and-a-half story, sixty-bed facility opened in 1855. After moving several times and facing growth in the population of Mobile, a new, $4 million, 250-bed facility, complete with air conditioning, opened on Spring Hill Street in 1952. The east wing of the earlier structure at this site, completed in 1908, supplied segregated hospital accommodations for Black patients. Accountable to the Sisters of Charity national order and not just to the local Mobile community board, questions would begin to surface about the appropriateness of Providence Hospital's racially segregated accommodations.

The establishment of the Mobile Infirmary (1910) marked the beginning of the transition in Mobile from hospitals serving a charitable mission for the poor into ones serving paying patients. Augusta Evans Wilson, introduced in the last chapter as a pro-segregation philanthropist, helped instigate the fund-raising drive that would result in the opening of Mobile's first voluntary, white-only facility. Opened in 1910, it included thirty-two beds, an operating room, and a laboratory. It would continue to expand over the next forty-two years. A new 285-bed facility was opened in 1952 on the eighty-acre former Oak Hill golf course site. Katherine White-Spunner, one of the first graduates of the Infirmary's nursing school in 1913, would go on to serve as its administrator for more than thirty years. She oversaw transition to the new site and the growth of the hospital from 70 to 520 beds. It became the largest, best endowed voluntary hospital in Alabama. White-Spunner grew with it, becoming a forceful presence. Even the most aggressive medical staff member cowered before her. The Infirmary took full advantage of the federal funding for hospital construction available after World War II raising concerns about its racially exclusionary practices.

Blessed St. Martin de Porres opened as a five-bed maternity service for Black patients in 1941. While the overall supply of adequate hospital care had lagged population increases and medical developments in Mobile, the gap was particularly acute for Black people seeking care. The Alabama State Department of Health released a report estimating that only 34 percent of the need for acute hospital beds for the Black population was being met.[10] Black physicians had no access to admitting privileges, worsening the problem. Four Sisters of Mercy served as the nursing staff for the five-bed facility and a Black physician soon replaced the original white obstetrician supplying maternity care. It was a token gesture. Building an adequate hospital to serve the broader hospital needs of Black patients and physicians was soon transformed into a national fund-raising effort. Bishop Fulton Sheen promoted it in his nationwide Catholic Hour radio broadcasts. Claire Booth Luce—politician, and wife of the founder of Time, Life and Fortune magazines —and others celebrity figures gave support to the cause. A city park was bought as the site. Bishop Sheen served as the speaker at the ground breaking ceremony noting that the "hospital was a national institution and not just one for the City of Mobile," revealing that contributions for its construction had come from every state in the union.[11] The resulting thirty-five bed hospital served Black patients, only about 15 percent of whom were Catholics. It would run with a biracial medical staff, the only one in Mobile and one of the few in the South. It was the first step in more fundamental and bitterly resisted hospital changes in Mobile.

The Hill-Burton Act

The post-World War II building boom that reshaped all these Mobile hospitals came from the funds made available by the 1946 Hill-Burton Act. All the ironies and opportunities for ending racial disparities in access to hospitals stood in stark relief in that Act and in the life of its main sponsor, Senator Joseph Lister Hill (D, Alabama). Born in Montgomery in 1894, he was the son of one of the South's most distinguished surgeons. He was named in honor of the father of aseptic surgery, Joseph Lister, whose techniques had yet to gain full acceptance among surgeons on this side of the Atlantic. Hill's father and Alabama's medical profession played a central role in shaping his ambitious legislative agenda. Hill would serve for forty years as a US Congressman and Senator sponsoring eighty major pieces of legislation. He was the archetypal Southern Democrat who became part of Roosevelt's New Deal coalition. While never crossing the Jim Crow divide on issues such as support for a federal lynching law that would have ended his political career, he supported Roosevelt's New Deal public works programs, rural electrification, and subsidies for cutbacks in agricultural production. Almost singlehandedly, he briefly convinced Alabama's overwhelmingly white electorate to vote in their own economic self-interest. As a result, Alabama gained the reputation of being the most liberal state in the South. Talk about Hill's potential as a presidential candidate, however, was silenced when he chose local political survival. He voted against all federal civil rights legislation and signed the 1956 "Southern Manifesto," pledging "massive resistance" to any federal court school desegregation orders that might follow the *Brown* Supreme Court decision. Senate Majority Leader Lyndon Baines Johnson was one of only three southern senators who did not sign the manifesto, earning southern enmity but keeping his presidential ambitions alive.

No legislation sponsored by Hill was more carefully crafted on the issues of racial segregation and medical autonomy or as profound in its impact as Hill-Burton. The Act provided a massive infusion of federal funding for hospital construction while undermining the momentum of the Truman National Health Insurance plan.

Hill-Burton offered two face-saving sweeteners for legislators concerned with supplying insurance access to hospital care: (1) facilities receiving funds were not allowed to discriminate on account of race, creed, or color and (2) had to supply a "reasonable volume" of free care to those in their community who needed care but could not afford to pay. The fine print of the nondiscrimination provision (section 662f) reads as follows: "such a hospital or addition will be made available to all persons residing within the territorial area of the applicant without discrimination on account of race, creed or color but an exception will be made in cases where separate hospital facilities are made available for different population groups if the plan makes equitable provision on the basis of need for facilities of like quality for each such group." It would enshrine in federal law a "separate but equal" provision in the special case of hospitals, the only such provision enacted in the twentieth century. Such provisions would soon be ruled unconstitutional by the *Brown* decision for public schools. It would, however, take another twenty years to mount a challenge to such segregation in hospitals constructed with Hill-Burton funds. Mobile's newly constructed hospitals, all built with Hill-Burton federal funding, would serve as a key test case in the implementation of the Medicare program. Alabama used the funds, as did some other southern states, to develop a "deluxe" version of Jim Crow that helped equalize racial disparities in access to hospital beds.[12] St. Martin de Porres hospital in Mobile was a part of that effort.

Once the Hill-Burton funds were distributed, however, federal oversight of the "separate but equal" and "reasonable volume" of free care requirements was nonexistent. The NAACP Legal Defense Fund challenged this in *Simkins v. Moses H. Cone Memorial Hospital*, 323 F.2d 959 (4th Cir. 1963). The decision held that "separate but equal" racial segregation in publicly funded hospitals was a violation of equal protection under the United States Constitution. This case, involving a similar pattern of Hill-Burton segregated financing of the hospitals in Greensboro, North Carolina, precipitated the inclusion of Title VI in the Civil Rights Act of 1964. Title VI prohibited the use of *any* federal funds in institutions or programs that discriminated based on race. (A similar legal challenge to the failure to enforce the "free care" requirement would follow, finally forcing the promulgation of federal regulations). The same LDF and legal aid lawyers who mounted these challenges would join in a struggle with Dr. Jean Cowsert to assure Title VI compliance in Mobile's hospitals with the implementation of the Medicare program. An irresistible force was about to meet an immoveable object.

PART III

Jean Cowsert, MD

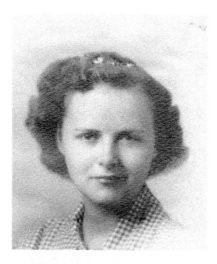

FIGURE 2. Jean Cowsert circa 1950, University of Alabama Medical School file. It is hard to avoid the penetrating stare from her medical school ID photo. Despite the staple holes in this small photo, her eyes still follow you. (UAB Archives, University of Alabama at Birmingham)

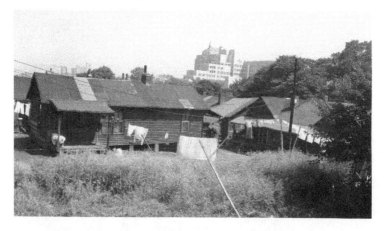

FIGURE 3. The University of Alabama Birmingham Hospital and medical school complex (circa 1958) loom over the low-income Black neighborhood surrounding it. Jean Cowsert received her early medical education and clinical experience here. Much of the neighborhood would soon be cleared to make room for the medical center's expansion (UAB Archives, University of Alabama at Birmingham)

CHAPTER SEVEN

Growing Up

PIECING TOGETHER A BIOGRAPHY of Jean Cowsert is a challenge. There are only a few people living, most in their nineties, who remember her. The rest of her story must be assembled from archival records—birth, death, and marriage certificates, census and school records, and a few newspaper clippings. She was born August 25, 1925, in Pensacola, Florida, next to Mobile along the Gulf Coast. She died at age 41 and is buried in the Pine Crest Cemetery in Mobile, Alabama. Her gravestone identifies her as "E. Jean Cowsert, MD." The Caduceus, symbol of medicine, is centered below her name between the date of her birth and death.[1] Her mother, Elsie Mae Williams was one of six children born to the family in Pensacola in 1896. Her father, James Hugh Cowsert, also one of six children, was born in rural Sarepta, Mississippi in 1887. The two were married at Elsie Mae's large family home in Mobile in 1916. According to a newspaper account, it was a festive and lavish social event.[2] By the 1920s the couple was living in Mobile and beginning to raise their two daughters, Elsie Jean and her older sister, Eleanor. Elsie Mae worked as a public-school teacher and James worked for the Life and Casualty Company of Tennessee, based in Nashville. James died in 1939 when

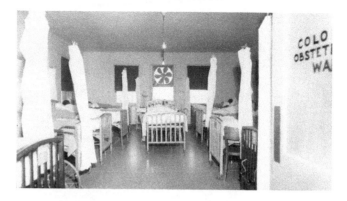

FIGURE 4. The UAB hospital "colored" obstetrics ward (circa 1960). Technically, it provided the best obstetric care available to Black women in the state. Many in rural areas lacked access to hospitals for financial reasons or Jim Crow restrictions. They relied on in-home deliveries by Black physicians and lay midwives (UAB Archives, University of Alabama at Birmingham).

Jean was fourteen. In 1942, Elsie Mae married Fred Hayes, proprietor of a garden center in Mobile.

Jean Cowsert shows up in newspaper archives, shedding some light on her childhood. Elsie Jean and her sister Eleanor were periodic contributors to "Aunt Jane's Letter Club," in the Sunday youth section of the New Orleans *Times-Picayune*.

> I am Eleanor Cowsert and am 12 years old, in fifth grade at school. I would be in a higher grade, but I had bad eyes and did not get to school at all until I was nine years old. . . . My younger sister Jean is nine years old. We would both like to join your letter club if you will have us. I am small for my age and Jean is large for hers, and some think we are twins, but I have dark hair and Jean is blond. I like to read and play quiet games, and everyone says we are as different as can be because if ever there was a "Tom boy" I guess Jean is one. She likes marbles, baseball, basketball and any outdoor game.[3]

Jean as a teenager continued to make contributions to Aunt Jane's

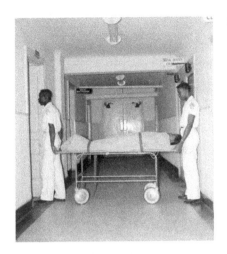

FIGURE 5. Orderlies with a stretcher pass a door labeled "white waiting room." State and local laws imposed strict separation of the races in the medical school complex. Federal financial pressure did not begin to bring the medical school Jim Crow barriers down in the South until around 1964 (UAB Archives, University of Alabama at Birmingham).

Letter Club. A movie review in 1940 reflected a growing predilection for action in the face of injustice that would shape the rest of her life.

PRIZE MOVIE SYNOPSIS: "WHEN DESTRY RIDES AGAIN"

This classic tale of the Wild West staring Randolph Scott and Kay Reynold takes place in 1891. Tod Jackson was moving westward as were many Americans during that period, when he stopped to see the Daltons. Yielding to their persuasions, he set up his law office in their city to help fight a crooked land company.

When he met Julie the girl Bob Dalton was to marry, he had vague misgivings about staying there. Finally, he could no longer constrain himself and confessed a love he found was mutual.

Meanwhile the Daltons had gotten in some trouble with the land company and had been arrested. When Bob returned from a trip he had taken, Tod was so busy with the trial that he didn't tell him of his love for Julie. After the trial began, Bob Dalton saw his brothers faced a "fixed" jury, so he drew his gun on the crowd. Under this cover the Daltons made a getaway from a peaceful, law-abiding life to one of crime. When Bob came back to take Julie away with him, she told him she loved Tod. He became furious with Tod and seriously injured him. Then he realized that Tod was a true friend and apologized. But the Dalton's had ridden their last mile. A posse was waiting for them and during the gunfight, the Daltons were all killed.

Tod continued his trip west, taking Julie with him. They kept the memory of the Daltons as true friends and peaceful upright citizens.

JEAN COWSERT
12 RICKLEY RD
MOBILE, ALABAMA[4]

The two sisters would go on to graduate together from Mobile's white-only Murphy High School in June 1941. They shared a love of music and took part together in the school's band, orchestra, and choir. Jean also received recognition as vice president of the school honor society Yo Tappa Kees and as a school auditor in her senior year. Six months later with the bombing of Pearl Harbor and America's entry into the war, the sisters would pursue different paths. Eleanor would marry and begin to raise a family. Jean would join the Army Signal Corps, serving as a radar and radio technician during World War II. The Army Signal Corps was the first to recruit members of the Women's Army Corps and recruited the highest percentage to their technical services as any branch in the Army. For the Signal Corps, mechanical ability and critical thinking skills were in high demand and gender was irrelevant.

Perhaps following in the footsteps of her mother, Jean took advantage of the educational benefits offered to World War II veterans and would get an undergraduate degree in education at the University of Alabama in 1948, earning a straight A average. The degree and the grades opened new opportunities. She applied and was accepted to the Medical College of Alabama. In 1954, the year of the *Brown* decision, she graduated first in her medical school class. She was one of two women graduating from a class of sixty. She had received straight A's in her first three years, only slacking off a bit on her surgery rotations with B's in her final year, perhaps reflecting her preference for the medical as opposed to the surgical side of medicine. Graduating at the top of her class or even just graduating as a woman from medical school was an unusual event at that time. She and five other female graduates of American medical schools who placed first in their class that year were honored at a special celebration at the Women's Medical Association meeting in Chicago. The event caught the attention of the women's page in the *Times-Picayune* and captured many of the assumptions about female roles that would take another couple of generations to begin to overcome.

SIX WOMEN BEST MALES AS MEDICAL SCHOOL OPENS

Meet the top women medical school graduates of 1954 . . . They are women who carried off top honors from their male classmates and were graduated head of their medical school classes . . . Not only did they top the men in class—some of them balanced long study hours with baby raising dishwashing and cooking for a husband . . . Dr. Cowsert was a radio and radar technician before entering the Medical College of Alabama. She was a straight A student at Alabama and won both prize competitions open to first-year students. She likes to raise Camellias and fish.[5]

Cowsert left Alabama for Detroit, completing an internship at Wayne County General. Like Mobile General, Wayne was part of a county-owned campus of facilities that had evolved from its County Poor House, founded in 1832. Just as other such county facilities, it was an attractive opportunity with plenty of "teaching material" for postgraduate medical training. Unable to adjust to the shifts in the organization and financing of medical care, Wayne County General closed in 1986.

Cowsert went on to a two-year residency in internal medicine at Detroit Receiving Hospital, followed by a two-year fellowship as an internist at the same hospital. Her presence at Detroit Receiving appeared in a photo in the *Detroit Free Press* on January 6, 1957, entitled "Women in White Line Up at Receiving." She appears in the photo with ten other women physicians in the stairway entrance to the hospital, most looking uncomfortable at being singled out for attention apart from their male colleagues. Detroit Receiving has since been renamed Detroit Medical Center and become part of a for-profit alliance affiliated with Wayne State and Michigan State Medical Schools.

Cowsert's stay in Detroit was sandwiched between the bitter race riot of 1943 and an even more destructive one in 1967. The 1943 race riot reflected the same conditions that produced the riot in the Mobile shipyards but on a larger scale. It was set off by the influx of about 400,000 poor white and Black residents from the South competing for housing and jobs. Thirty-four deaths, mostly Black victims and mostly from police interventions, resulted. Almost 6,000 federal troops were used to restore order. But the 1967 riot proved worse than any since the draft riot in New York City during the Civil War. It left forty-three dead, 7,200 arrested, and four hundred buildings destroyed. A police raid on an illegal, afterhours Black "blind pig" club touched off the riot in an increasingly racially tense city.

For Black people escaping Jim Crow in the South, Detroit was not much of an improvement. They faced all forms of housing discrimination, blocking their exodus from the city and crowding them into a ghetto. The relocation of the auto plants to the suburban areas surrounding Detroit increased Black disparities in employment opportunities. Detroit's police force was 93 percent white with a tendency toward violence against the city's growing Black population. The Detroit area even had a growing Klan presence.

Orville Hubbard, mayor of Dearborn from 1942 to 1978, became a national symbol of Northern racism, perhaps even rivaling the notoriety of Birmingham, Alabama's Bull Connor.[6] Dearborn was one of the segregated white suburbs ringing Detroit, well supported by a tax base that included the Ford Motor Company. Hubbard made no effort to hide his stranglehold grip that controlled Black exodus from Detroit. He fought the development of a low-income housing project in Dearborn in 1948. Hubbard was concerned that it would become a "Black slum." His aides passed out leaflets encouraging residents to "keep the Negroes out of Dearborn." In 1956 he became a national figure when he told an Alabama newspaper that he was "for complete segregation, one million percent."[7] In 1965 the federal government unsuccessfully charged him with conspiring to violate the civil rights laws when a Dearborn house was vandalized by a mob stirred up by rumors that the house had been sold to a Black family. He was a strong supporter of George Wallace in the 1968 presidential campaign. Hubbard's oft repeated sound bites certainly strengthened the impression that he and his city did not welcome Black neighbors. During the 1967 riots he issued the order to Dearborn police to shoot looters on sight. That he was elected mayor of the town for fifteen consecutive terms or 36 years suggests that the white citizens of Dearborn were not that welcoming either.

Rosa Parks, icon of the Montgomery bus boycott, had suffered her own indignities. White opponents of the Montgomery civil rights movement had long memories. Parks faced economic retaliation and telephone threats. She lost her job at the Montgomery Fair department store, her husband lost his job as a barber at the Maxwell Airforce base, and other options for employment in Montgomery disappeared. She and her husband migrated to Detroit in 1957 to find work, overlapping with Cowsert's post medical school training there. Parks continued her civil rights efforts as a staff member for Detroit congressman John Conyers between 1965 and 1988. Conyers worked for the passage of Medicare in 1965, introduced legislation in every session to create a single payer universal health system, proposed legislation to create a slavery reparations commission (later designated as H.R. 40, referring to the Union's Civil War promise of "40 acres and a Mule"), and introduced a bill to make Martin Luther

King's birthday a national holiday (finally signed into law by President Reagan in 1983). Symbolism came easy, concrete results harder. Parks died in 2005 at age ninety-two. A bronze statue of her was installed in 2013 in the US Capitol's National Statuary Hall. She sits as she did on the Montgomery bus, the only statue not linked to a state and the first full-length statue of an African American in the Capitol.

Detroit, for all its limitations, served as a center of resistance to the excesses of Jim Crow in the South. Activists in the "Negro District" of Detroit or "Black Bottom" served as a center of resistance first to the fugitive slave laws and later in the Jim Crow era to the rendition of Black citizens to face dubious charges and questionable justice in Southern states up through the 1950s.[8] Sympathetic Michigan judges and politicians helped.

For Cowsert, however, the stark segregation of health care in Detroit matched that of Mobile but was more dishonest. An "understanding" helped city funds subsidize the operations of small private hospitals set up by Black doctors unable to get privileges at the white ones. While the care provided by these under-resourced facilities was often abysmal, it saved money for the city by not forcing a major capital investment in the expansion of Wayne County General and keeping its white medical staff and patients segregated.[9] "I lost my faith," Cowsert later confessed to a friend in Mobile.[10]

In 1959, Cowsert returned to Mobile to set up a practice in internal medicine and began to blossom. She became a welcomed addition to the medical staff at Providence Hospital, operated by the Daughters of Charity of St. Vincent de Paul. One of the hospital's administrators later reflected on her contribution.

We loved her. She was an excellent physician and person. The first woman doctor I knew that wore dresses instead of pants like a man. She wore pearls and was very good looking. She won the approval of the medical staff in a male dominant field. The male doctors began referring patients to her. The doctors recognized her competence and commitment, liked, and respected her. She became president-elect of the medical staff in 1965, the first woman to hold such a position in the Mobile Metropolitan area. She was a very good physician and loved her work as a doctor.[11]

Sister Mary John, a nurse at Providence and a patient of Cowsert's, had nothing but praise.

> She was a brilliant diagnostician. She diagnosed me with acute appendicitis. The surgeon disagreed and wanted to wait and see. The next morning the appendix almost burst. The surgeon later wrote her a letter of apology for his mistake. Another time I called her because I didn't feel well. She told me to come in immediately because she could tell from my voice I was suffering from an allergic reaction to medications.[12]

Praise for this strong, opinionated female newcomer was not unanimous. The influential pathologist at the Mobile Infirmary, Dr. Earl Wert, recalled her differently.

> She was a strong, abrasive person. She did not get along with the other doctors and was not part of the crowd that socialized together. Providence at that time was for the "have nots" and the Mobile Infirmary was for the "haves" so I can imagine how she felt. She was not a popular person.[13]

She was not, however, the kind of person who seemed to worry much about being socially or professionally popular. In 1966, as the new medical staff president at Providence, she plowed ahead with a medical audit process, an intrusion into their hospital practice certain to annoy some of her colleagues. It focused on assuring a degree of accountability among medical staff members and preventing profitable but unnecessary procedures. It was a concern that had been raised earlier by younger, specialty-trained physicians in the city after World War II.[14] "We have become the first hospital in Alabama to enter into The Professional Activity Study—Medical Audit Program sponsored by the American College of Surgeons, American College of Physicians and the American Hospital Association," announced Cowsert at the press conference.[15] The project at the time included more than six hundred hospitals, accounting for more than four million discharges a year operating in forty-four states, the District of Columbia, Puerto Rico, Canada, and Australia. Cowsert went on, "In other words, the chart of every patient admitted to Providence Hospital will be compared with the others in PAS-MAP. (Professional Activity Study–Medical Audit Program). We can see if our treatment is as good as in these other hospitals." The data represented about 12 percent of all discharges in the United States and 18 percent of those in Canada. Sister Andrea, the hospital's administrator, recommended it to the hospital's board. The Board approved it Cowsert noted, "to improve the level of care here through the education of all the staff. . . . It's the most valid hospital statistical program of its type in the country. I don't think we fully realize the full benefits we can obtain from them yet." Such oversight was not something many physicians welcomed. The program ushered in a new era of more standardized treatment and payment for hospital care. It helped bring an end to the unnecessary surgery at the hospital. Cowsert understood the value of such efforts in improving patient care and, during her tenure as chief of the medical staff, she served as a forceful advocate.

Portraying her as just a statistical nerd, however, does not do her justice. She was entranced by the complexity of the more humane, ethical, even spiritual side of medicine and shared it at a health care conference for administrators of the Sisters of Mercy's hospitals, later published.[16] She wrote, "Into this program of statistics and reality I come to you as a dreamer, bringing my dream to share with you for a time. I hope that you will take it with you and let it grow, so that some not-too-distant day we can return here and hear the statistics of a program based upon its translation into reality."[17] She then launched into her dream of a program for improving the community-wide health of those connected to the Order, with the spiritual, holistic, and preventative focus that have become more common to more contemporary notions of population health.

While she may not have spent much time currying the favor of her Mobile male physician colleagues, she was hardly the isolated malcontent that some of them portrayed her as. She moved in with her mother, Elsie Mae and her stepfather, Fred Hayes. Her mother had a heart condition and had been hospitalized several times. Hayes operated a nursery on the premises of their home and Jean shared his interests as a gardener of flowers. He was hard of hearing and a bit frail as well, so the shared living arrangement helped Jean look after them both. Both enjoyed having her join them and followed her evolving medical career with interest.

Providence Hospital became her medical home and the nuns that ran it soon became an extension of her family. They served as a much-needed nurturing antidote to her Detroit experiences. Jean's home with her parents became a welcoming gathering place. She loved to fish and soon persuaded her new friends to join her on fishing trips. She chartered the boat, and her mother packed the sandwiches for these outings. Their disembarking from the harbor grabbed the attention of those in the other boats: "We were still in our 'flying nun' outfits and we had to tie them down to keep them from blowing us out of the boat."[18]

On one of these fishing expeditions, Cowsert climbed down to the cockpit to pay the charter captain. She stumbled and was knocked unconscious.

We rushed her back to Providence and stayed with her all night, waking her every several hours as you're supposed to do. At six or seven in the morning she woke up on her own and asked, "how do I take instruction to become a Catholic?" She had been thinking about it for a long time. For her it was a sign that she should do it, just as St. Paul had fallen from his horse and knocked unconscious only to hear the words of Jesus and become converted. I told her to tell Sr. Andrea, the administrator, and she would arrange for a priest to instruct her. I covered for her when her parents called when she was taking instruction. She didn't want to tell her mother because it would upset her, until she was sure. She took profession of faith and Holy Communion in January 1964.[19]

The storm clouds over Jim Crow health care in Mobile were gathering. Step by step, without becoming fully aware, Cowsert was coming closer to the center of the storm.

CHAPTER EIGHT

An Irresistible Force Meets an Immovable Object

A STORM HAD BEEN GATHERING but Mobile seemed so well protected. Its hospitals had all benefitted from the influx of federal dollars for new construction and expansion provided by the 1946 Hill-Burton Act without relinquishing any control of their destiny. Hill-Burton's principal sponsor, Senator Joseph Lister Hill (D, AL) had made sure to include a provision in the law that protected Jim Crow. For white doctors in Mobile, it seemed the best of all possible worlds. Incomes of physicians were rising, receiving help from the growth of the postwar economy, private health insurance, and medical knowledge. Nationally organized medicine had used the growing deference accorded its practitioners to defeat Truman's national health insurance legislation and seemed certain to assure the protection of its interests in the future.

Most community hospitals, however, were struggling to cover the costs of medical advances. Only the Mobile Infirmary, focused on a white, more privately insured, and affluent population, seemed to be on an upward trajectory. The members of the Mobile County

Medical Society, however, were well insulated from financial struggles of individual hospitals. They were free to choose where they admitted their patients.

The 1954 *Brown* decision had unleashed massive resistance against
the desegregation of public schools in Alabama blocking even modest changes. The desegregation of private hospitals and medical services was beyond anything that seemed possible. No one could have
expected what would take place over the next decade.

Hospitals and the Civil Rights Movement

Hospitals were invisible during the height of the civil rights movement
in Alabama. The Montgomery Bus Boycott, the Freedom Rides, the
lunch counter sit-ins, and the peaceful marches for enfranchisement,
all surrounded by violence, got the headlines. Few protests related to
hospitals took place and even fewer were covered by the press. But
quietly, the pressure for hospital desegregation kept growing. Even
when desegregation was initiated, it was rarely acknowledged. Hospital boards and administrators feared a backlash that would affect
their census and their financial viability, as well as potentially provoke
ire from their patients. It was easier just to pretend that it had always
been integrated and its segregated history just disappeared. Perhaps
one of the most remarkable losses of this institutional memory took
place with Moses Cone Hospital in Greensboro, North Carolina.

Greensboro, North Carolina, the seed bed for the student nonviolent lunch counter sit-in movement, was also the seed bed for the
hospital desegregation movement.[1] The town had three hospitals that
had all received Hill-Burton funds. The racial makeup of these facilities was like that of Mobile's. There was Wesley Long, a white-only
community hospital; L. Richardson, set up for Black-only care; and
Moses Cone Memorial, the largest and most well-resourced facility.
Except for a few limited specialty services not available at the Black

hospital, Moses Cone was for white patients only. Black physicians only had privileges at L. Richardson, the Black hospital.

George Simkins, local NAACP president and dentist in Greensboro, was frustrated by the lack of access to hospitals. Simkins recruited Black physicians to join him in legally challenging Moses Cone and Wesley Long. The legal brief argued that by accepting federal construction funds as part of a state Hill-Burton hospital planning process, the two hospitals were no longer functioning as private entities. They had become part of a "state action" that violated the due process clause of the Fifth and the equal protection clause of the Fourteenth Amendments of the Constitution. Their protracted legal battle gathered momentum when Attorney General Robert Kennedy joined in support of the Simkins position in the federal courts. For the attorney general to join in attacking a federal law rather than defending it was unusual. However, President Kennedy's civil rights legislation, deliberated in the House in fall 1963, included a similar provision (Title VI) that prohibited the use of any federal funds for racially discriminatory purposes. Simkins and the Greensboro physicians prevailed in the 4th Circuit Court and the Supreme Court quickly declined to review it, letting the 4th Circuit's decision in Richmond, Virginia stand. This result not only forced Long and Cone to desegregate but added an aura of judicial inevitability to the inclusion of Title VI in the Civil Rights Bill, which faced a lengthy filibuster by Senate Dixiecrats in the spring of 1964.

The Civil Rights Act of 1964 (Pub. L. 88–352, 78 Stat. 241, enacted July 2, 1964) did not directly address hospitals. Most assumed that the Simkins decision would require protracted legal battles with every segregated hospital in the country that had received Hill-Burton funds. Other than Hill-Burton funds at that time, most hospitals received little federal aid. While Title VI prohibited racial discrimination in programs and activities receiving federal funds, it was deliberately vague about what that meant or how it would be enforced, if at all. Most insiders assumed that Title VI just represented cosmetic window dressing to placate Congressman Adam Clayton Powell (D, NY) who, with the guidance of the NAACP, had the annoying habit of regularly proposing a similar amendment to every appropriations bill. Except for major teaching hospitals that received federal funds for training and research, the federal government had little other financial leverage over private hospitals.

Federal financial leverage over the nation's hospitals, however, was about to change. Johnson's landslide victory over Barry Goldwater in November 1964 opened the opportunity to pass the Medicare and Medicaid legislation in 1965. Federal payments to hospitals from these programs would soon account for as much as 50 percent of hospital revenues. Nobody mentioned the Title VI implications of this in the debate over passage. Most assumed that, just as the *Brown* decision had proved for public schools, Title VI would have an inconsequential impact on hospitals. The door, however, had been opened and the rising tide of the civil rights movement did the rest. The Medicare and Medicaid funding supplied leverage to quietly transform most hospitals almost overnight. Unlike with the *Brown* decision and public schools, there was no such thing as "all deliberate speed." If hospitals wanted to serve as a Medicare provider, hospitals had to follow all the conditions in their provider contract. Six thousand hospitals did so by July 1, 1966, the day that the Medicare program began. Perhaps the most racially segregated institutions in American society had become one of the most integrated almost overnight. The Simkins decision for Moses Cone Hospital had begun a radical transformation of hospitals all over the United States.

Alvin Blount, MD, had joined George Simkins in the lawsuit and helped recruit five other Black physicians in Greensboro to join as well.[2] He had already broken the color barrier becoming the first Black chief surgeon of a MASH unit during the Korean War.[3] Blount could shut out the mayhem surrounding the bunker and focus only on the wounded soldier on his operating table. His calm, gentle demeanor commanded respect and he received a Korean War service medal. His story also became incorporated in a novel and movie that later became a long running popular television series M*A*S*H (the series excluded the Black surgeon supposedly for "historical accuracy" reasons but more likely to avoid restricting its adoption by local TV stations in Southern states). As a result of the Simkins suit, Blount also became the first Black surgeon to join the medical staff of Moses Cone Hospital. In 2016 at age 94 he was the only surviving plaintiff and was still seeing a few elderly patients in his primary care practice. A Black surgeon and president of the medical staff, Dr. James Wyatt, made a point of acknowledging Blount's service and this history at his last meeting as president. Wyatt first acknowledged the lengthy service of an elderly white physician on the medical staff to the Greensboro community. This drew polite applause from the audience. He then acknowledged Dr. Blount and the role he had played in desegregating hospitals in the country. It was like a bolt of lightning. It drew a five-minute standing ovation. Except for Dr. Wyatt, no one on the medical or in the hospital's management had been aware of this history.

This precipitated a special event shortly afterward that included Dr. Blount, family members, key community leaders, and the staff of the hospital. Terry Akin, CEO of Moses Cone, addressed Blount: "It seems to me, and to our medical and dental staff, that we needed to take the opportunity to apologize for our role in this chapter in our history and to honor those individuals for challenging us to be the best of ourselves and for their foresight and courage in changing America." The hospital donated $250,000 to a scholarship fund honoring Blount and the other plaintiffs, which provides support for minority students seeking health care careers. It is administered by the Greensboro Medical Society, one of many local Black medical societies across the country that played a role in the hospital desegregation struggle. A highway historical marker next to the hospital was unveiled shortly afterward, honoring the plaintiffs and their role in changing the nation's hospitals. Too few events or efforts to commemorate desegregation activists have taken place.

Blount passed away after a brief illness shortly after the celebration at Moses Cone Hospital. His family marked his passing with a quiet event at the small Episcopal church next to the North Carolina A&T University campus that had served earlier as the organizing center for the lunch counter sit-in movement. "My life is my memorial," he had told his practice manager. "No big casket or cemetery plot either – cremation —just be sure I'm dead before you burn me." His life included caring for wounded soldiers in Korea, feeding arrested Dudley High School students during the sit-in demonstrations, and caring for his seven children. He sewed up a teddy bear for his youngest son, who was inconsolable because it had lost an arm, with the same concentration and concern as the GIs he treated in a Korean MASH unit.

Mobile's hospitals became prime targets for desegregation efforts in 1964 because of the Hill-Burton funds they had received and the Simkins decision. John LeFlore and his Nonpartisan Voters League had sent complaints concerning the hospitals to John Quigley, Department of Health, Education and Welfare (DHEW) Assistant Secretary responsible for civil rights. Michael Meltsner, the attorney at the NAACP Legal Defense Fund who had managed the *Simkins v. Moses Cone* case, assisted in the preparation of these complaints in anticipation of bringing lawsuits. Mobile's hospitals refused to budge.

But Jean Cowsert did. Providence Hospital broke ranks and desegregated their patient floors. Only a handful of hospitals across the South had done so and all paid a heavy price. At Providence, it began with a symbolic gesture by Cowsert. According to Sr. Bernice, the administrator:

She integrated our hospital by admitting her house maid to a white floor and that started the whole thing. No one dared stop her. We almost went bankrupt. We lost a lot of patients. Dr. Cowsert would try to get hers admitted to Providence but many white patients of hers insisted on being admitted to the Infirmary where she also had privileges.[4]

One of the Providence hospital's nurses at the time had similar recollections:

It was a difficult transition for everybody. Many of the white patients refused admission and went to the Mobile Infirmary instead. The census dropped down. The administrator and some of the nurses from the North were resented. Whites that did come brought their own pillows so they wouldn't have to sleep on one Blacks had. Many tried to change rooms or move into a private one if they had to share one with a Black patient. We were an older facility and had few private rooms to accommodate such transfers. The Blacks didn't like the change either.[5]

Except for a few principled (or fool hardy) cases such as Providence, voluntary desegregation by hospitals was not going to work. Only John LeFlore and the Nonpartisan Voters League seemed pleased with what Providence had accomplished and what few other hospitals in the South had dared to do. In a letter to John Quigley at HEW on August 13, 1965, LeFlore reported, "We are pleased to advise you that Providence Hospital now projects a picture which indicates that it is in compliance with Title VI of the Civil Rights Act. The hospital in our opinion has pursued a determined policy in almost all areas to meet the demands of Title VI."[6]

Medicare, signed into law by Lyndon Johnson on July 30, 1965, however, changed the stakes for hospitals and for those seeking to desegregate them. The new federal funding for hospitals was massive and would account for as much as 50 percent of hospital revenues. Title VI of the 1964 Civil Rights Act prohibited "discrimination on the grounds of race, color, or national origin" in any programs and activities receiving Federal financial assistance. If you violated this prohibition, you ceased to be eligible for the funds. Title VI, however, provided no guidance on how this "discrimination" would be documented or the prohibition against it enforced. As of February 1, 1966, a newly created Office of Equal Health Opportunity in the Public Health Service with five full-time equivalent staff was responsible for certifying that 6,000 hospitals were fully compliant with Title VI in four months. How could it be anything more than mindless paper compliance, just checking a few boxes on a form and mailing it in?

We may live in unusual times but not any more unusual than those in 1966. In summary, five conditions shifted the odds of such a gargantuan task.

1. **Timing:** 1966 marked the height of the Civil Rights movement. The 1964 Civil Rights Act, the 1965 Voting Rights Act and, with the support of many of the same activists, the Medicare and Medicaid legislation had been passed in 1965. Local Jim Crow laws and conventions regarding public accommodations were collapsing and there was a growing acknowledgment among local leaders in the South of its inevitability.

2. **Leadership:** An unusual combination of individuals occupied key positions in the federal bureaucracy. Wilbur Cohen and Robert Ball, career technocrats, were trusted by legislators of *both parties* with the morass of details involved in managing Medicare's implementation. They were never directly challenged because it was correctly assumed by all parties that they knew more about how to get this important program off

the ground than they did. John Gardner, Secretary of DHEW, a public intellectual with a doctoral degree in psychology, a former private foundation president, and the only Republican in Johnson's cabinet, could cast a spell on almost everyone with whom he interacted. He never mentioned race, segregation, discrimination, or inequalities but argued for upholding the constitution, the rule of law, and treating everyone and all organizations consistently and fairly. Johnson was mesmerized by him. Gardner transformed his request for the directors of the HEW agencies to donate "volunteers" to staff the hospital Title VI certification effort and absorb the cost into an act of moral responsibility and patriotism. Gardner had built a "field of dreams" and, despite the dangers, had no trouble getting passionate civil rights activists volunteers to play in it.

3. **Money:** The hospitals needed it. Costs were rising and about half their patients were over the age of sixty-five. Most had no insurance and could not afford to pay for hospital care out of pocket. Medicare was a lifeline that could transform institutions teetering on the edge of bankruptcy into profitable, growing enterprises. They were mostly voluntary private hospitals, not public ones, which were less insulated from local political pressures. The decision to desegregate was in the hands of a privately constituted self-perpetuating board whose primary responsibility was to protect the assets of their non-profit enterprise and not to local political leaders. No matter what hospital administrators and board members personally felt about racial integration, they were not about to refuse to cooperate and lose out on the funding that would now flow to their competitors. Many just quietly went about making the necessary accommodations without it even appearing in the local news media.

4. **Standards:** The basic standard was clear and precise: race could play no role in how the hospital operated. That meant everyone had to use the same exits and entrances, waiting areas, cafeterias, and parking lots. Patients had to be assigned to rooms randomly on a first-come, first-serve basis and there could be no matching by race. Hospital medical privileges and staff hiring had to make every effort to compensate for past exclusion of Black applicants. Patients could be referred to as Mr., Miss., or Mrs., or by their first names, but everyone, without regard to race, had to be referred to in the same way. There could be none of the traditional pattern of referring to white patients respectfully by title and Black patients by the first name or other disrespectful titles such as "boy." The Southern defense of de facto segregation continued to be that people should be allowed "freedom of choice." The response of the federal Title VI enforcers in 1966 was, "Yes, you have freedom of choice, you have the freedom to choose any provider, but if you choose one that participates in the Medicare program you cannot be treated differently by race. That is what the constitution and law say, period."

5. **Transparency:** Some facilities that, in current parlance, thought they could "fake it until they made it" had a rude awakening. Nothing escaped the notice of local civil rights activists and the Black hospital workers closely aligned with the movement. Some facilities tried what was called "The HEW Shuffle": move the patients around in advance of the inspection visit so the hospital appeared integrated and, after the inspectors left, reshuffle them back. A phone call from a Black hospital worker or local activist brought the inspectors back in a less tolerant mood. Nothing like this could be hidden.

Given these five conditions, one might conclude that the "mission impossible" was not enforcing Title VI compliance but circumventing it. The hospitals in Mobile, Alabama, however, proved to be the ultimate test of such a conclusion.

The Ultimate Test Case

In the fall of 1965, it looked as if little was going to happen using Medicare Title VI certification to desegregate the nation's hospitals. The Hill-Burton complaints submitted by LeFlore to DHEW concerning Mobile's hospitals remained unresolved. Over the summer and fall of 1965, the NAACP Legal Defense Fund, the Medical Committee for Human Rights and the National Medical Association had submitted collectively more than three hundred similar Hill-Burton Title VI complaints against other hospitals that remained unaddressed.

The Medicare and Medicaid Act became law on July 25, 1965, with the Voting Rights Act following closely on August 6. For Johnson, however, these triumphs paled in the face of the Watts riots that began August 11 and sank him in despair. With a history of racial abuse, Los Angeles police officers attempted to arrest a Black man for drunk driving in the Watts neighborhood. Inflamed by allegations of police brutality, it produced six days of rioting, thirty-four deaths, and forty million dollars in property damage and required almost fourteen thousand California national guard troops to suppress. Amid the riots, John Gardner became the new secretary of HEW. Johnson, responding to the Watts riot white backlash, began an effort to bury civil rights enforcement efforts out of sight, deeper into the federal bureaucracy. Many civil rights activists concluded that this was an effort to make them disappear.

On September 24, 1965, Johnson summoned Vice President Humphrey, who had served as the lead in coordinating federal civil rights activities. Johnson announced that he was removing Humphrey from that responsibility. He had decided that all civil rights enforcement matters would be decentralized and administered by the agencies and officials responsible for specific programs. In a cruel twist of the knife, Johnson demanded that Humphrey present this reorganization plan as his own, signed, enthusiastic recommendation.[7] Gardner, the new secretary of HEW, was left to figure out what this meant for the implementation of the Medicare program that would begin on July 1, 1966.

A disastrous event added to the uncertainty about how civil rights enforcement would be managed in the new Medicare program. A well-researched Title VI complaint concerning de facto segregation in the Chicago public schools had been submitted by Chicago civil rights groups on September 30, 1965, to Francis Keppel, Commissioner of Education at HEW. It demanded that Keppel hold up the release of $32 million in new funds to the Chicago Public School System.[8] Commissioner Keppel sent a letter to the Illinois officials indicating that the Chicago Public School System was in "probable noncompliance" with Title VI and that these issues had to be resolved before these new funds would be released. In a face-to-face meeting, an enraged Mayor Richard J. Daley confronted Johnson. Johnson called an immediate evening meeting, summoning Gardner, Keppel, and other key federal officials to the White House. Domestic advisor to the president Joseph Califano called Mayor Daley to let him know the money would be coming. Wilbur Cohen flew out to Chicago the next day to complete the arrangements and Keppel was relieved of duties as Commissioner. It did not auger well for Title VI enforcement by lower-level officials in the federal bureaucracy. Throughout the autumn the inaction in managing the Hill-Burton complaints matched the inaction in addressing the Chicago public school complaints. Just urging voluntary compliance was not going to work either, as demonstrated by the difficulties that attended Providence hospital's desegregation in Mobile.

On December 7, 1965, John Holloman Jr., MD, president of the National Medical Association (NMA) and the Medical Committee for Human Rights (MCHR), the two organizations that had submitted the bulk of the Hill-Burton complaints, requested an appointment with Secretary Gardner. A report was also submitted at the same time by the NAACP Legal Defense Fund to the secretary. It highlighted the importance of Medicare Title VI compliance, urging HEW not to "throw away a superb opportunity to end racial discrimination in Southern hospitals."[9] Despite confusion concerning the scheduled meeting, Gardner was already working from the same script. On December 14, 1965, he circulated a memo to every part of HEW outlining the staffing plan that would be used to enforce Title VI. Stripped of its deliberately vague bureaucratese, the memo basically said HEW is a civil rights enforcement agency and every component of HEW will be responsible for providing the staff and budgets to support the critical mission of enforcing Title VI in the implementation of the Medicare program. Is this what Johnson had in mind in decentralizing civil rights efforts? We will never be sure, but it soon became too late for him to stop it.

Two new components of the HEW bureaucracy emerged over the next two months. A small group, which would over time evolve into the Office for Civil Rights in the Secretary's Office, coordinated and assured consistency in policies across the different components of HEW. Derrick Bell Jr., its legal counsel, was recruited from the NAACP Legal Defense Fund. He would go on to a distinguished career as a law professor, authoring many books. He is credited with being one of the foundational thinkers of "Critical Race Theory," now an object of rage by some right-wing spokespersons. The actual Title VI certification of hospitals for Medicare was managed by the Office of Equal Health Opportunity (OEHO), which began to take shape in the Public Health Service in February 1966. Temporary volunteers from the different parts of HEW, who would staff the office and conduct most of the field inspections, began to be assembled in March. Marilyn Rose, one of the other few females that graduated from Harvard Law School in that same class with Ruth Bader Ginsberg, served as in-house legal counsel. On loan from the Justice Department, Rose would be directly involved in the Mobile hospital desegregation battles with Dr. Jean Cowsert.

The volunteers began to arrive, and the survey and inspection plan took shape. The plan followed the general outline of the inspection process used by civil rights groups in generating Title VI Hill-Burton complaints against hospitals. A series of two-day workshops prepared the trainees. The first two workshops were in an auditorium at the Center for Disease Control in Atlanta in early April. Those conducting the training were key people from the Medical Committee for Human Rights (MCHR), the Student Nonviolent Coordinating Council (SNCC), and the Southern Christian Leadership Conference (SCLC). A unique form of regulatory capture had taken place, not by powerful drug, insurance, or medical lobbies, but by the civil rights movement.

No one was sure it was going to work. In regions of the country where no Jim Crow laws had ever existed, Title VI certification of the hospitals was on schedule. In the South it was not. Sometime in April, Peter Libassi who directed the civil rights group in Gardner's office had a meeting with presidential advisor Joseph Califano at the White House.[10]

"How is the hospital certification effort coming along." Califano asked.

"It's going smoothly in most parts of the country. The only problem is that almost none of the hospitals in the deep south are going to be eligible to get Medicare funds when the program begins." Libassi replied.

Califano did a double take, "What do you mean?"

Libassi explained how the certification worked. Hospitals had to be FULLY compliant with ALL the requirements—not all deliberate speed "progress" would be acceptable. It appeared that it was the first time he had heard this. As far as the White House had been concerned, Medicare's implementation was on autopilot, not something they needed to deal with. Libassi now had Califano's attention.

"Let me get back to you." Califano said.

He never did, but the Title VI certification process was now on the White House's radar. They started paying attention to the weekly reports concerning hospital progress in Medicare certification forwarded from the OEHO. On May 6, Libassi sent a memo to Califano indicating that in the twelve Southern or border states less than 50 percent of the hospitals had been certified for participation in Medicare and some had not even responded to the original request for information.[11] On May 19, Douglass Cater, the other White House staff member responsible for domestic policy matters, sent a memo to the president that urged a rethinking of the Title VI approach to desegregation. He argued that it was a "faulty instrument which Congress added to the Civil Rights Act just to keep Adam Clayton Powell from adding it to every piece of legislation that came along."[12] A White House staff memorandum from the director of Emergency Planning to the president on May 23 reflected growing concern about whether the Title VI certification bluff was really going to work with the Southern hospitals.

> For practical purposes compliance with Title VI for hospitals will be complete for all hospitals except Alabama, Louisiana, Mississippi, and South Carolina. Alabama and Mississippi are probably not to be greatly improved . . . Governor George Wallace is now trying to get Southern governors to a meeting and is encouraging hospitals in his own state to refuse compliance. Where there are gubernatorial elections, his conduct poses a real problem.[13]

President Johnson, now fully engaged, turned up the heat on the southern hospitals. In a Rose Garden ceremony on June 3, he received the Award of Merit from the National Council of Senior Citizens. Busloads of seniors from every state arrived to participate in the event. Johnson urged them to go back to their local communities and help "alert your hospitals of the requirements of the law, particularly the nondiscrimination requirements of Title VI. Encourage them to meet those requirements."[14] On June 15 key leaders of hospitals and medicine were summoned to a meeting at the White House to get a final briefing on the Medicare program. The attendees included a Who's Who of the nation's hospital and medical leaders. Dr. Jean Cowsert, as chief of staff of Providence Hospital in Mobile, was among them. After the update by key staff, Johnson made his pitch. In the film footage of the meeting, Johnson marches past Cowsert to the podium and wastes no time getting to the point.

> Now we know there are going to be problems. One of them arises with compliance with the laws of the land, specifically the Civil Rights Act. In some communities older people may be deprived of medical care because hospitals fail to give equal treatment to all citizens, and they have discriminatory practices . . . The Federal Government is not going to retreat from its clear responsibility and what the members of Congress have written into the law. And I hope you will not retreat either.[15]

According to Libassi, Johnson then departed from his well-polished prepared script. He raised himself to his full height, fixed his glasses, leaned over the podium, and stared sternly at the assembled leaders: "We ain't going to lock the barn door after the hoss has been stolen. We're going to desegregate the hospitals!"[16]

At the time of the White House meeting on June 15, *none* of the hospitals in Mobile had been certified to receive Medicare funds. HEW officials, perhaps not wishing to single out Providence Hospital for more of the difficulties it had already experienced in desegregating, was not certified either. Altogether 327 hospitals, including the four in Mobile, awaited Title VI clearance on June 30, 1966. On July 1, 1966, Providence, Mobile General, and St. Martin de Porres got Title VI approval to become Medicare providers. The Mobile Infirmary did not. The Infirmary became a test case in a bitter protracted battle that would shape the future of health care under the Medicare and Medicaid programs. Either at the White House meeting on June 15 or shortly before, Dr. Cowsert was recruited to play a secret, key role in that battle. She became its key fatal casualty.

Criminal Conspiracy or Freedom of Choice?

The battle over Title VI certification of the Infirmary became the ultimate Jim Crow zero-sum game with no possibility for compromise. For the staff of the Office of Equal Health Opportunity, it was a matter of assuring the integrity of the certification process. For the Mobile Infirmary, it was a matter of protecting the integrity of the physician-patient relationship. Individual physicians and patients, the Infirmary argued, should have complete "freedom of choice" over where patients would be referred for hospital care and should not be subjected to any outside pressure.

This battle of wills began with Jean Cowsert's efforts to desegregate Providence in 1965 and culminated in the decision not to certify the Infirmary for Medicare participation on the first of July 1966. A secret collaboration had evolved between Cowsert, LeFlore, and key staff in the Office of Equal Health Opportunity. Cowsert was also a member of the Infirmary's medical staff. At the Infirmary medical staff's regular meetings, she had learned of the plan, supported by many members, to circumvent the desegregation of this historically white-only hospital. In theory, the plan would still enable the Infirmary to be Title VI certified for Medicare. Its members would just continue to refer their Black patients to the other hospitals in the city. The referral patterns of physicians ultimately determine how separate and unequal medical care is whether in 1966 or today. The Infirmary's medical staff, just as with most hospitals at that time, was a separate organization not under the direct control of the hospital's management or board. The hospital had no direct control over where its medical staff members chose to admit patients. The hospital could claim, almost with a straight face, that it admitted and treated every patient referred to it by its medical staff members without regard to race. The hospital could thus comply with Title VI in principle while in practice remaining lily white. Since physicians had been specifically exempted from Title VI compliance under the physician payment component of Medicare (Part B), they faced no financial repercussions for this racially discriminatory behavior.[17] Cowsert was appalled by the cynical intent and so was the Office of Equal Health Opportunity. If hospitals could remain segregated in this way and still be certified to receive Medicare, the whole purpose of the Title VI certification effort would be undermined. If the Infirmary succeeded, its tactic would spread quickly to many other hospitals, making a mockery of the whole effort to assure racially equal treatment. The Infirmary thus became a test case for the argument that a hospital's management and board had a responsibility to prevent such behavior among its medical staff members and, if it failed to make a good faith effort to do so, it could not be certified as compliant with Title VI.

From the perspective of members of the Infirmary's medical staff supporting the racially selective hospital referral scheme, their professional responsibility to their patient was at stake. The physician, in consultation with his patient, they argued, had the absolute right to choose where they should be admitted. In Mobile, it was a time-honored precedent, reflecting the open nature of staff privileges at its different hospitals and the proximity of the facilities.

Physician referrals have always been a delicate matter full of land-mines. Fee splitting between physicians referring to surgeons in the 1920s was considered unethical. It became a major focus of the American College of Surgeons' hospital reform effort. Fee splitting was grounds for refusing medical privileges to physicians or terminating them. Many more recent complicated financial arrangements between referring physicians and hospital specialists have been ruled illegal. In the absence of Jim Crow law prohibitions, more subtle pressures on physician hospital referral patterns in many Northern metropolitan areas produced almost the same segregated conditions as in Mobile.

> In America doctors got their hospital staff appointment every year or two or, at most, every three years. While there is something approaching tenure if you have been on the staff for say, twenty-five years without a blemish, doctors are not always courageous, and they sure knew that in some of these hospitals with the ghetto encroaching that it would be sacrilege to admit a Black.[18]

Professional hospital administrators in all regions were also shaped by the American College of Surgeons hospital standardization program and shared a similar organizational culture to those at the Infirmary. In an article in *Hospitals* after the passage of the 1964 Civil Rights Act, Everett Johnson, the Chief Executive Officer of Methodist Hospital in Gary, Indiana, anticipated the concerns expressed by some of the Mobile Infirmary physicians.

> The law creates a fundamental problem for patient care in general hospitals . . . To legislate that physicians and hospital staffs must ignore emotions in patients arising from any cause is to amend the historical right of medicine to make the patients wellbeing its most important concern. When patients have predetermined convictions

on racial matters, efforts to force change in them at the time of illness can be detrimental to their medical care. Because the rendering of medical care is the hospital's responsibility, it must be its primary consideration. Difficulties will arise in the implementation of the Civil Rights Act. It is unfortunate that sick people will have to face these problems.[19]

Each party, whatever the motives, claimed the moral high ground, creating a long, bitter, battle. The highest stakes battle in the Medicare hospital desegregation campaign began in Mobile on July 1, 1966. Providence, Mobile General and St. Martin de Porres were cleared to receive Medicare payments. Cowsert, without any protection against retaliation nor any possibility for compensation had become OEHO's whistleblower. She was their "mole" and most essential intelligence asset. Cowsert kept OEHO informed of developments and soon alerted them to another loophole the Infirmary's medical staff had found. Medicare would pay hospitals not certified to receive funding for "emergency admissions." Suddenly Medicare patient admissions to the Infirmary all became coded as "emergencies." Cowsert brought this to OEHO's attention, and these payments were stopped. Indeed, other southern hospitals had resorted to this gambit and these practices were curtailed as well. The battle against all these holdouts intensified. The Infirmary's census dropped. An entire wing with more than one hundred beds had to be closed but the hospital's board and management refused to budge. Cowsert provided a list of Infirmary staff members that were the ringleaders of the racial boycott to OEHO. OEHO then requested the hospital provide admission statistics for each of these staff members by race. The Infirmary's management refused.

In December 1966 that refusal drew a flurry of support for the hospital's management from the Alabama Hospital Association, Mobile County's Medical Society, and the Infirmary's own medical staff.

All insisted that the doctor and patient must have complete "freedom" in hospital admission choices. The doctor-patient relationship in arriving at that decision, they insisted, was sacrosanct. The hospital had no right to interfere with such decisions or pressure the physician or patient about that choice: "Members of the medical staff and medical society notified Robert Nash and Phil Lee of HEW that they do not intend to dictate to their patients the hospital where they will be treated ... they allow complete freedom of choice in such matters to patients."[20] "We protest the attempt to misuse the services of the doctors of Mobile County as a tool of pressure to achieve a social goal, no matter how important it may seem to its proponents."[21] An editorial appeared in the *Mobile Register*: "Never happy unless throwing its weight around against somebody or something, the Lyndon Johnson Great Society racial integration by force bureaucracy continues to use the Mobile Infirmary as a whipping boy by refusing to certify it for the admission of Medicare patients."[22] Many hospitals had tried to use the "freedom of choice" argument to justify the continuation of segregated accommodations *within* their facility, but this had been relatively easy to manage. No one, and certainly not a hospitalized sick person, was likely to cross even an invisible color line. The fear of retaliation was just too great. Hospitals had always been responsible for decisions about the assignment of new patients to rooms. This was different. It was challenging the decision of patients and their physician about which hospital to be admitted to and that, for many physicians and patients, touched a raw nerve.

The pressure for a settlement intensified. Governor Wallace described the denial of payments to the Infirmary as "not only heartless but the most immoral act I can imagine" and demanded a Congressional hearing. In a telegram to HEW Secretary Gardner, Wallace noted that "it's inconceivable that a government agency would allow old people to suffer and possibly die because of some illegal demand made on the part of HEW (e.g., to admit more Blacks to the

Infirmary). Wallace said that "it was his understanding that physicians leave up to the patient which hospital he or she is to enter, and I wonder if you are going to start telling doctors all over the country that they must assign their patients as you direct them rather than in the manner they think best."[23] The anger and frustration from the Mobile Infirmary's board and management no doubt rose on news from its rival Providence Hospital. Providence, benefiting from the infusion of Medicare dollars and patients while taking advantage of Hill-Burton federal matching dollars, announced on December 21, 1966, plans for a major expansion to add 140 beds.[24] The political pressure generated by scathing local press coverage and contacts with congressional representatives by Infirmary and medical society representatives had become intense. HEW's top officials decided to take the decision out of the hands of OEHO and try to negotiate an accommodation. Dr. Leo Gehrig, deputy surgeon general, was sent to Mobile to try to work past the impasse. Gehrig had been sent there just before Medicare's implementation to meet at the Mobile Civic Center with more than one hundred community leaders, including Mayor Joseph Langan as well as hospital, medical, and Chamber of Commerce representatives. He had to explain why the certification of Mobile's hospitals had been held up, so he was generally familiar with the issues.[25]

Before he left for his early January visit to Mobile, Gehrig met with OEHO's director Robert Nash and its legal counsel Marilyn Rose. They shared all the information they had on the case. Nash and Rose also supplied contact information for their mole, Jean Cowsert. He could get updated intelligence from her, but this had to be done with care since she would face certain retaliation if her role in this standoff became known. Gehrig flew to Mobile in early January. His visit included a more than five-hour conference with Mobile Infirmary officials. Members of its board of trustees and medical staff executive committee attended. Asked by the press if there had been any progress in resolving the matter, Gehrig was noncommittal, "some progress had been made, since it was important to explore issues."[26] E. C. Bramlett, the Infirmary's administrator, was equally vague. "We are talking. We are working together, I am certain everything will work out in the end."[27] No one seemed to have budged. Yet Gehrig's assignment, objected to by the OEHO staff, was to bring this controversy to as quick and as quiet an end as possible. Gehrig promised there would be continued discussions with the Infirmary in the next week. All the Infirmary had to do was to keep the pressure on. The Mobile County Medical Society did its part. They published an advertisement in the paper pleading with Mobile citizens to write political leaders in Washington. The medical society argued that federal officials, by holding up Medicare certification for the Infirmary, were attempting to "dictate doctor-patient relationship matters in violation of medical ethics and customs" and they would never abandon the practice of allowing patients to choose their own hospital.[28] It was a distorted framing of the issue, but it produced the intended result. A letter to President Johnson was forwarded to Gehrig for response. That response was published in the *Mobile Register* and held up for ridicule in an editorial.

Anxious to bring an end to the Infirmary problem, Gehrig returned to Washington with a plan. He met with Nash and Rose about his proposal, which sounded to them like total capitulation. Far worse, they learned that Gehrig had ignored well-established protocols. His conversation with Cowsert was by phone from his Mobile hotel room through the hotel's switchboard. Nash and Rose were aghast. Federal representatives working on civil rights issues in the South at that time had to assume that such calls were monitored. Even temporary transfers involved in the inspections, as one observed later, were careful to use public phones. A doctor familiar with the situation at the time stated: "We knew for sure that if we talked from a motel it would be listened to. We knew that from what could be heard in the background and what people said to us afterward, that we were listened to."[29] Gehrig had blown Cowsert's cover.

According to Rose, a few days later, Robert Nash, the Director of OEHO, got an early morning call from E. C. Bramlett, the administrator at the Mobile Infirmary, telling him that Cowsert had been found dead. The Administrator knew of her relationship with the Office, or he would not have called and, if he knew, others did. Was it his way of suggesting that the death was suspicious and should be investigated or was it, as one native of Mobile concluded, a veiled threat (e.g., "Don't mess with us!)"?

To review the limited evidence again, the fatal bullet had apparently been fired from Dr. Cowsert's own revolver. No one in Mobile, however, took the notion that the death was an "accident" seriously, as the pathologist at the Infirmary and the city's part-time coroner had concluded. A noise, apparently caused by a rock being thrown through her kitchen window the night of her death, had interrupted Cowsert as she was writing a letter to the Sister in charge at Providence urging arrangements be made to assure that all the Sisters got regular medical checkups. It was a letter written by a person fully engaged in the practice of medicine and unphased by the desegregation controversy swirling around her. It was not the kind of letter one writes as an immediate prelude to a suicide.

Nor was the coroner's conclusion plausible that it was a result of an accident, where she had tripped and fallen, causing the gun to be discharged into her chest. It was a clear night with a full moon in familiar surroundings for a person familiar with guns and how to use them. The pendant around her neck had been broken and there were bruises on her neck. Mobile, however, seemed eager to put Cowsert's death behind them and the coroner's ruling that the death was an "accident" came less than two days later. Her mother, medically frail and hospitalized at the time of her death, did not want any further investigation. "Enough bad things have happened," she said. What "bad things" was she afraid of? Had she been threatened? Most of the evidence related to Cowsert's death—records of the Mobile Police Department's investigation, the autopsy report, records of the requested FBI investigation, OEHO's own files, and correspondence related to the event among local leaders—either disappeared or was destroyed.

Several weeks after Cowsert's death, the Mobile Infirmary administrator, E. C. Bramlett, got a call from Senator Hill letting him know that the battle was over and formal notification would follow. The Infirmary had been approved for "provisional" Title VI clearance. It was now eligible for Medicare payments, retroactive to February 1, 1967. In the notification that followed, OEHO identified some modest improvement in admission statistics. The *Mobile Register* headline read, "Medicare Fight Won by Hospital."[30]

The federal Medicare civil rights offensive came to an end. On June 28, 1967, the home of the civil rights leader John LeFlore who had led the effort to desegregate Mobile's hospitals, was firebombed. On July 1, 1967, the Mobile Infirmary received full Title VI clearance. Six months later the occupancy of the Infirmary had reached 93 percent and it was completing plans for a six-story addition. OEHO was shut down soon after this. Its functions were absorbed into a centralized Office for Civil Rights in the Secretary of HEW's Office. This made it more easily accountable to the Congressional subcommittees responsible for its funding, all controlled by Southern legislators. The Office for Civil Rights in HEW never got the budget and staffing to continue the site inspections provided by the volunteers that assisted with Title VI certification during Medicare's implementation. Both racial disparities in referrals for specialized diagnostic services and treatments for heart disease, cancer, and other diagnoses and the debate over the hospital and medical staff's role in addressing such disparities continue with no awareness of these long-forgotten events. No one has since been bold enough to propose publicly that disparities in a physician's referral patterns be grounds for discipline or terminating hospital privileges. Cowsert's death and her righteous battle disappeared even from local memory.

CHAPTER NINE

Cowsert and the Cages

JEAN COWSERT'S DEATH ended the civil rights offensive. Medicare scrapped plans for Title VI inspections of nursing homes. Physician payments remained exempted even from paper Title VI compliance until the passage of the Affordable Care Act in 2010. Federal support of regional planning to assure equitable geographic access to services ceased in the 1980s. Progress in eliminating racial disparities stalled.

Despite a century of improvements, racial disparities in pandemic death rates widened between the nation's last two major pandemics. There were no racial differences in death rates from the influenza pandemic of 1918.[1] This helped at that time to refute the scientific racism arguments of innate Black inferiority.[2] During the first year of the COVID pandemic that began in 2019, Black age-adjusted COVID hospitalizations were 2.85 times higher than for whites, intensive care unit admissions were 3.17 times higher, and hospital death rates were 2.58 times higher.[3] A century of medical progress produced pandemic indicators of racial differences worse than those that have been typically used in the past to argue for urgent corrective action.

Higher rates of poverty were a major contributor to the COVID racial disparities, not just disparities in medical care. More whites than Blacks now face all the health disparities resulting from poverty, including a second-class, Jim Crow–era system of health care. Cowsert and other medical leaders at that time recognized this. Fourteen months after Dr. Cowsert's death, a bullet fired at Martin Luther King on the balcony of the Lorraine Motel in Memphis ended a broader effort to eliminate poverty. King envisioned a natural interracial alliance that would end poverty. His death helped set poverty in stone in the richest nation in the world.

It was not the first time such coalitions have died in this country. In the post-Reconstruction era in Alabama, a coalition of Black Belt plantation owners and Birmingham industrialists controlled state politics partly through fraudulent manipulation of ballots. They shared an interest in low taxes, minimal government services, control over their labor force, and restrictive voting that would by more legal means support these interests. The Bourbon coalition, as it was called, feared a populist alliance between poor whites and Blacks. In 1900, 180,000 Alabama Black people could still vote. Federal court rulings and the successful implementation of white supremacy electoral "reforms" in Mississippi, South Carolina, Louisiana, and North Carolina showed the way to legally eliminate the threat of a populist takeover. Bourbon electoral control could be assured through a proposed new constitution that would eliminate the Black and poor white vote. The 1901 Constitution passed by a narrow, probably fraudulent margin.[4]

Conservative ideologues are just as nervous today as the white ruling elite was when they pushed through Alabama's 1901 Constitution. The "chasm" between most Trump supporters and social justice reformers is an illusory one. Face to face, there is much less hate than what the gun advocates, racist ideologues, and fundraisers try to stir up. Most Trump supporters don't want anybody touching the Medicare and Social Security benefits they and their families rely upon.

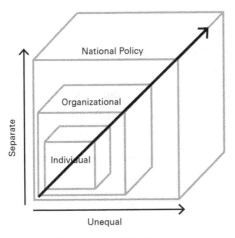

FIGURE 6. The structure of Jim Crow health care, 2023

Just after the presidential election in 2020, a Black group demanding that the Albany legislature raise the minimum wage crossed paths with an angered group of Trump supporters protesting the certification of Biden's victory. When the white protesters in the MAGA hats learned what the Black protesters were demanding, they shook hands and joined their protest.[5]

At the height of the civil rights era Medicare came close to desegregating health care and creating a single universal standard. Its success touched off similar successful initiatives eliminating discrimination based on sex and disability. Borrowing from Medicare's Title VI provision, Title IX of the Education Amendments of 1972 prohibited federal funding of higher education that discriminated based on sex. It transformed the universities almost overnight just as the similar provision had transformed hospitals. The Americans with Disabilities Act of 1990 followed. It prohibited federal support of institutions that discriminated against persons with disabilities and similarly transformed public spaces.

Standing in the way of ending disparities in health care as well as poverty, however, are the Jim Crow cages illustrated in Figure 1 (see

Preface). The log jam will most likely be broken by universal health care. Public opinion polls support it. Universal care would finally end the separate market of health care services for the poor and the selective referral system that Dr. Jean Cowsert fought against that perpetuates disparities. It will be a difficult struggle more akin to the nineteenth-century abolitionist struggle against slavery than that of the 1960s civil rights era. The "new abolitionists" face the more entrenched twenty-first-century replacement—poverty—not slavery.[6]

Today the Jim Crow cages are less imposing, as portrayed in Figure 6. The arrow once forcing their enlargement now begins to shrink their size. Many picked up where Dr. Cowsert left off, determined to put an end to the legacy of slavery and Jim Crow. A diverse, loosely connected new abolitionist movement has done the shrinking. Their work began with attempts at a full recovery of memory about a shameful past. As Jerry Mitchell, an investigative reporter in Jackson, Mississippi, who has done more to open unsolved murder cases of the civil rights era than anyone, says, "I have been told again and again to let the past be. But I have found that a true account of a painful past does more good than murky optimism, We must remember to point our compass towards justice. We must remember and then act."[7] In Alabama, that recovery of memory has been led by the press in an internet merger, AL.com, that has captured national attention. Kyle Whitmire of this group won a Pulitzer Prize in 2023 for his work exposing how Alabama remains caged in its white supremacy past and how the "Alabamification" of America cages the nation.[8]

The Cold Cases

Fear served as the foundation of the Jim Crow system. Failure to hold people accountable for acts of terror perpetuates that fear. Though 4,084 Black people were lynched in the South between 1870 and 1950, less than 1 percent of the cases ever led to criminal convictions.[9] The track record in prosecuting hate crimes through the civil rights era was little better. The death of Emmett Till, a fourteen-year-old boy visiting relatives in Mississippi in 1955, sparked the beginning of civil rights era struggles. The cold cases, still fresh in the memories of Black families, cast a shadow. They fuel a distrust of white institutions that is hard for medical providers to overcome. That distrust contributes to fewer preventive services and referrals for needed specialized care.

In 2008, Congress passed almost unanimously the Emmett Till Unsolved Civil Rights Crime Act (Pub L. No. 110–344, Stat. 3934 [2008]). The Act authorized the Department of Justice to designate a deputy chief of the Civil Rights Division to coordinate the investigation and prosecution of such cases. A supervisory special agent in the FBI's Civil Rights Unit was assigned to investigate them. The Justice Department was given the authority to coordinate these efforts with state and local law enforcement officials. For fiscal years 2008 to 2018, Congress authorized the Justice Department to spend $10 million a year and the FBI $2 million a year.[10] Only a fraction of this authorization was ever appropriated. Yet the issue could not be dropped either. The Emmett Till Unsolved Crime Reauthorization Act of 2016 (Pub. L. No. 114–325, 130 Stat. 1965 [2016]), approved almost unanimously, extended this effort for another ten years.

The Department of Justice's task under this Act is to develop a complete list of such cases, open investigations of them, and prosecute as many as possible. The fifty-six field offices of the FBI were directed to identify cases that might warrant inclusion. Other potential cases were solicited from the National Association for the Advancement of Colored People (NAACP), the Southern Poverty Law Center (SPLC), and the Urban League. The Justice Department also conducted outreach to community groups, law enforcement officials, universities, and the national media to solicit additions to the list. As of March 21, 2021, 132 cases have been opened for review. Of the 119 fully investigated and resolved, ten were referred to states for possible prosecution, two were federally prosecuted, and the remaining 107 closed without prosecution.[11]

The odds of successful federal prosecutions were minimal. Almost all the cases predated the 1968 Shepard-Byrd Act that made hate crimes a federal offense. Murder prosecutions fall under the authority of states. People cannot be prosecuted for doing things that were not crimes when they were done. Southern legislators successfully blocked passage of almost two hundred antilynching bills in Congress between 1882 and 1968. In 2022, the Emmett Till Antilynching Act, making any bias-motivated murder a hate crime and thus a federal offense, was enacted into law with almost unanimous bipartisan support. Prior to this, federal prosecution of lynching was limited to the Reconstruction era-Fourteenth Amendment prohibition against states denying individuals equal protection and due process. Since most of the civil rights era race-based murders were committed by private actors (such as Klan members), federal authority depended on demonstrating a connection to state actors (for example, that a murder was committed with the assistance of police).

Time imposed even greater barriers. People cannot be prosecuted for murders if they are already dead. If all those with any direct knowledge of the event are dead, it is also almost impossible. Memories and records disappear with time and, as a rule, civil rights era cold cases stay cold. Two exceptions illustrate what it took to break that rule. One was the finally successful prosecution of the three surviving perpetrators of the church bombing in Birmingham that resulted in the death of four girls.[12] The other was the conviction of the Klan leader responsible for the murder of civil rights workers James Chaney, Andrew Goodman, and Michael Schwerner in Mississippi.[13] Seared into the national conscience, these two cases could never be closed. The case of Jean Cowsert's death, its possible connection to her efforts as a civil rights whistleblower unknown, was ruled an accident in two days and closed like so many others.

The Civil Rights and Restorative Justice project (CRRJ) at Northeastern University Law School tries to pick up where the Emmett Till Unsolved Civil Rights Crime Act leaves off. The project's goal is to recover an accurate history and try to use it to remediate the ongoing damage to the families of victims and to society. The CRRJ project lent their assistance to the Cowsert investigation.

Professor Margaret Burnham created the CRRJ project in 2007 reflecting a long career related to civil rights era cold cases and concern for the ongoing trauma faced by the families of victims.[14] She worked as a lawyer for the NAACP Legal Defense Fund in the 1970s, successfully defended Angela Davis, and became the first Black woman to be appointed as a judge in Massachusetts. Burnham also headed a team of outside counsel and law students that resulted in one of only two successful federal prosecutions reported by the Justice Department under the Emmett Till Act. The case involved the murders of Charles Moore and Henry Dee by Klansmen in Franklin County, Mississippi, in 1964. The murder conviction of James Ford Seale was upheld in 2010. The Klan members made the mistake of murdering their victims in a national forest that gave the federal government authority. Professor Burnham was appointed in 1993 by South African president Nelson Mandela to serve on an international human rights commission to investigate alleged human rights abuses of the African National Congress (ANC). It served as the precursor to South Africa's Truth and Reconciliation Commission that followed and her own efforts with the CRRJ project. She was also appointed in 2022 by President Biden to the Civil Rights Cold Case Records Review Board. The board's purpose is to help expedite the release of government archival materials related to such cold cases to help with the CRRJ project and related ones.

The CRRJ project's own archive now includes records on more than 1,100 possibly racially motivated homicides from fourteen Southern states occurring between 1930 and 1970. It provides a learning experience in civil rights investigations for law students, a way to assist the families of victims to achieve closure, and as a resource for researchers. The archive now includes seven completed cold cases that took place in Mobile County.[15] Most were originally but unsuccessfully brought to the attention of authorities by John LeFlore while he was head of the Mobile NAACP. One in 1943 resulted in the shooting of a uniformed soldier by a bus driver. The soldier, trying to return to the Brookley Air Force Base before curfew, expressed impatience when the driver stopped to chat with a friend. The incident sparked a bus boycott that resulted in banning bus drivers from carrying firearms. Two cases involved men killed by police officers and another two by shop keepers, all with conflicting accounts of the events. One case was dropped because of the reluctance of relatives to participate further in the investigation.

One final Mobile case illustrates what can best be hoped for in such efforts. In 1948, fifty-three-year-old Rayfield Davis was returning from his job as a janitor on the Brookley Air Force Base. He struck up a conversation with Horace Miller, a twenty-year-old white mechanic. The two got off the bus together. Davis invited Miller to join him for a beer at his home. Miller was offended by this impertinence that violated Jim Crow rules. Davis suggested that considering President Truman's proposed reforms, Black people would soon be equal to whites. Enraged, Miller beat Davis to death and left him in a drainage ditch. Miller, accompanied by a lawyer, confessed to the crime and signed a written confession. The resulting grand jury refused to indict him and a subsequent effort by the local NAACP to reopen the case failed. Davis's surviving family was recently contacted by the CRRJ. This resulted in a memorial ceremony, the laying of a memorial at the site, and a street renamed in Davis's honor. Miller's granddaughter participated in an apology for her still-living grandfather's act, and a spokesperson for Davis's family prayed for and forgave Miller. Some of the dark shadow of this senseless act was lifted from surviving family members.[16]

The Project's assistance in the Cowsert case involved three law students making phone calls to anyone that might have information about the case, combing the internet for documentation, and following up with subsequent leads. The students' and my own efforts produced the following conclusions:

1. **All of those on the initial list of "persons of interest" as potential suspects are dead.** That list, provided by John LeFlore in his correspondence to the Medicare Title VI compliance unit in the Public Health Service in December 1967 included twenty-six members of the Mobile Infirmary's medical staff most active in opposing the admissions of Black patients. Cowsert presumably assisted in supplying these names. All would have certainly learned of her betrayal and possibly more about the subsequent events surrounding her death.

2. **All of those involved in the original investigation of her death are dead.** Listed in the original story in the *Mobile Register*, Detective Captain Joseph Birch of the Mobile police force headed the investigation assisted by three other detectives, a sergeant, a police officer, and an identification officer. Most died prematurely in an occupation not noted for long life expectancies. In 1997 the author was able to interview Earl Wert, MD, the coroner who conducted the autopsy. He died shortly afterward. Even so, his recollections of the autopsy examination were vague and, according to him, the record of it had been

destroyed in a fire. One of the law students was able to contact Wert's son who recalled discussing the case with his father and his uncertainty concerning the cause of death.

3. **Only a few living friends, family members, and coworkers could be contacted.** Sister Bernice Coreil, who helped direct Providence Hospital while Dr. Cowsert was on its staff, now serves as senior executive advisor to the president of the Ascension Health System. She was interviewed by phone as well as Sister Mary John Code, a nurse responsible for the obstetric floor and emergency room during that time. Three physicians who knew her were also interviewed in 1997. Cowsert's sister's son, now a coroner in Kentucky, was also contacted. He recalled her fondly and was pleased with the effort to give her some belated recognition.

4. **Archival records related to the death are now almost non-existent.** A Freedom of Information Inquiry of the FBI investigation into Cowsert's death requested by Marilyn Rose, legal counsel to the Office of Equal Health Opportunity, indicated that there was no record of such an investigation. A Freedom of Information Inquiry of the Department of Health and Human Services indicated that, as required by federal regulations, all records of the Office of Equal Health Opportunity not classified as public documents had been destroyed. The Mobile Police Department reported that they had no record of the investigation and the record of the autopsy apparently had been destroyed in a fire. Local historian Scotty Kirkland observed that such missing records were not unusual.[17] He was unable to find City records of either the investigation or autopsy into the death by lynching of Michael Donald in 1981 in Mobile. The Donald case was a much higher profile, more recent one,

but Kirkland had to rely on a copy of the autopsy report in federal court records. Though US congressman Jack Edwards was in regular correspondence with the board president and chief executive of the Mobile Infirmary, no correspondence in the files was turned over to the University of Southern Alabama archive during the key six months when HEW refused to approve them for Medicare funds. Even the file on Jean Cowsert at Providence Hospital, kept on all physicians that have served on its staff, was unusually bare, according to Sister Bernice Coreil. The local television station WKRG-TV, on air since 1955, had done an interview with LeFlore concerning the refusal to certify the Mobile Infirmary for Medicare in December 1966 and certainly covered the story of Cowsert's death at the end of January 1967. Unfortunately, in 1976 the station converted from film to videotape and old film coverage went out with the trash. The only official acknowledgment of her death that has survived is a Memorial Resolution passed by the Medical Society of Mobile County in February 1967 acknowledging that "On 29 January 1967 death unexpectedly took our beloved friend and colleague Dr. Elsie Cowsert; and WHEREAS during her lifetime Dr. Cowsert wholeheartedly and with unusual dedication participated in the welfare and health of this community. . . . Her ability, accomplishment, ambition, gentleness, and devotion were an inspiration to all."[18]

The CRRJ Project's interest in the Cowsert case, however, led to it being officially added to the Emmett Till cold case investigation list in 2022. It is now one of twenty-six open cases being investigated under the Emmett Till Act by the Department of Justice. For the first time the Cowsert case has all the resources necessary for a full criminal investigation.[19] An FBI agent in their Mobile office and a civil rights attorney in the Department of Justice head the investigation.[20] Cowsert's surviving family members, delighted by the attention that the case has finally received, have been interviewed. The UAB archives have been searched for related material. All the resources used in the completion of this book have been shared with the investigation team. The list of closed cases includes seven involving the deaths of white persons and two Black physicians. Dr. Cowsert is the only white person and only physician among the still open cases. Perhaps more can be uncovered about the circumstances surrounding her death.

Most likely, the Department of Justice will conclude that no federal prosecution is possible and the case, just as almost all the other Till cases and our own efforts on behalf of Dr. Cowsert, will be closed. Was Cowsert's death an accident, suicide, or murder? Neither an accident nor a suicide makes any sense. The evidence leans toward the conclusion of OEHO staff who worked with her at the time that it was a murder.[21]

If one were writing this as fiction, it would be an easier story to tell. The motive was clear and the means available. Her medical colleagues at the Infirmary, those listed as leaders of the effort to block Black referrals to the hospital, were most certainly enraged by her betrayal and possibly knew more about the events surrounding her death. It would have been an indirect, hard to trace, careful, and calculated form of revenge. The Klan had a visible presence at the time in Mobile and it would have been easy to pass along word of this betrayal to them. Even "Dynamite Bob" Chambliss, responsible for the church bombing that killed three young girls in Birmingham, regularly made freight deliveries there from Birmingham. With most such Klan events, the purpose was to terrorize rather than kill. Late Saturday night, the perpetrators might also have been well fortified with alcohol. The stone thrown through the kitchen window did not elicit a call to the Mobile police since Cowsert probably assumed, as most did at the time, that there was too much overlap between members of local police departments and the Klan. Cowsert, not one to be easily intimidated, went out to confront them. A struggle ensued, resulting in the fatal discharge of her weapon.

Backlash

A backlash after Dr. Cowsert's death undid many of the reforms in the organization and financing of care that had helped desegregate and reduce disparities. The infusion of federal dollars with Medicare, Medicaid, and other programs originally came with the requirement that, not only would those services be racially integrated but that they would also be geographically distributed equitably to reflect community needs. Standardized payments through the Medicare program helped level the playing field for providers in poor as opposed to affluent communities. A planning and Certificate of Need process was supposed to assure that new programs and facilities would be equitably allocated to communities to reflect need.

Most of the "reforms" in the organization and financing of health care that have taken place since Dr. Cowsert's death never considered and often exacerbated the segregation and inequities in access to care. The discriminatory "impact" has been easy to document. Providers just made the rational business decision and moved facilities and services from communities where they could make less money to those where they could make more. The racially discriminatory "intent," well disguised as a preference for free markets, privatization, and reducing the role of government, was almost impossible to prove legally. Undoing the discriminatory impact calls for "reverse engineering" of the financial incentives or the planning process to achieve more equitable outcomes.

Even the standardization of payment in Medicare was soon "reformed" to work against its intent. The shift to Diagnostically Related Group (DRG) payment for acute care hospitals in the 1980s shortened hospital stays and shifted care to more segregated home and community-based settings. The shift was supposed to make care more efficient and save money, but the per capita cost of hospital care remained the highest in the world.

Inpatient hospital care became more segregated consequently. Hospital occupancy declined. In Mobile and in many other cities, this led to a conversion to all private rooms. Random assignment of patients to semi-private rooms had been a key test of Title VI compliance during the implementation of Medicare.[22] It was implemented with little opposition by patients or hospital officials, rare even in hospitals in the deep South. There was less evading of the desegregation guidelines than suggested by Northern critics. As one Southerner responsible for Title VI certification observed, "if they tell you they will do it, they do it. These are people that come to a full stop at stop signs in the middle of the night."[23]

Even Carraway Methodist Hospital in Birmingham, Alabama, with a history as a white-only facility like the Mobile Infirmary, complied with the guidelines. In the grip of Jim Crow resistance, Carraway refused to treat James Peck, a white Freedom Rider beaten at the bus station by Klansmen in May 1961. In 1968, however, floor nurses complied with the new Title VI guidelines and confronted an enraged patient and Klansman, "Dynamite" Bob Chambliss. According to Title VI guidelines, a Black male patient had been randomly assigned to Chambliss's semi-private room. Swearing, Chambliss threated to blow up the hospital as he had the church if that "n . . . ." wasn't removed from his room.[24] Chambliss was threatening them by admitting his role in the murder of four little girls in the bombing of the Sixteenth Street Baptist Church. The nurses, refusing to be intimidated, arranged for his discharge and called his family to get him. That took courage. An atmosphere of fear still gripped Birmingham. The FBI, reportedly, blamed the abandonment of their investigation into the church bombing on the assumption that getting a jury to convict the perpetrators would be impossible. While the nurses reported his verbal admission of guilt to local police investigators, they shrugged it off. It took the justice system another decade to convict and send Dynamite Bob to prison for life. Yet the floor nurses still concluded that "there was no such thing as freedom of choice" in these matters. Hospitals in the South, despite all the changes, remain substantially more integrated than in other areas of the country.[25]

Nursing homes also soon faced similar payment pressures that resegregated care. Resource Utilization Group (RUG) payments to nursing homes in the 1990s provided financial incentives to shift care away from institutional settings to home and community-based ones. However attractive the idea sounded in the abstract, it increased racial segregation and disparities in care. Just as with hospitals, a "level playing field" in access to home and ambulatory services across racially and economically segregated neighborhoods has never existed.

Market based "freedom of choice" insurance reforms of both the Medicare and Medicaid programs produced a system that racially resegregated patients by plan. "Freedom of choice" had always been a code word used to argue against integration, just as it was used to block the racial integration of admissions to the Mobile Infirmary. HEW's position on Title VI at the time of Medicare's implementation was that patients participating in a program financed with federal funds do not have that constitutional choice. Medicare and Medicaid patients now do, and care is now increasingly racially separate and unequal. Economic and racially selective referrals by physicians, the battle Dr. Cowsert fought at the Mobile Infirmary, are now built into the system.

Prescription

The level of trust patients have in their providers of care and the patterns of care that result is shaped by the larger environment that care takes place within. Other things being equal, the more segregated and unequal a society, the more segregated care and the greater health disparities will be. Voluntary initiatives of individuals and health facilities help but require legislative backbone.

Doing the right thing is always much easier if it pays. For example, soon after Dr. Cowsert's death, almost all the medical practices in Mobile eliminated their segregated waiting rooms. No law forced them to do this. Most physicians, just as the hospitals, wanted the Medicare money. "There has always been something more important than race," activist-historian Howard Zinn observed of this period.[26] It was usually money. Black elderly patients now had real bargaining power and were willing to use it. Consequently, Mobile Infirmary admissions of Black patients grew and soon matched their representation in the larger service area's population. Overall hospital segregation and racial health disparities in Mobile and Alabama are now less than in most northern metropolitan areas and states.

Many health care providers have begun their own informal version of a truth and reconciliation process like that of post-apartheid South Africa. As Desmond Tutu, chairperson of that process in South Africa, observed, "forgiving is not forgetting; it's remembering—and the remembering part is particularly important; Especially if you don't want to repeat what happened."[27] In 2008 the president of the AMA delivered a formal apology to the NMA. Included with that apology in *JAMA* was a detailed report jointly produced by the two organizations documenting the AMA's history of past racially discriminatory behavior.[28] Similar apologies from historically white state medical associations, including Mississippi's, followed. As described in Chapter 8, Moses Cone hospital in Greensboro, where the legal battle began to desegregate the nation's hospitals, apologized in a ceremony for its prior history of excluding Black physicians.[29] Other hospitals have made similar apologies.

An informal process of house cleaning is now also underway. In

2020, the University of Alabama, as requested by its Board of Trustees, removed the name of Josiah Nott from one of its buildings. This Civil War Era Mobile physician was an influential proponent of scientific racism and credited with helping to found the University's medical school. In a similar gesture that same year, the Association of American Medical Colleges (AAMC) removed the name "Abraham Flexner" from it most prestigious award, for excellence in medical education. Flexner, the "father" of modern medical education was also the author of racist opinions that no longer reflected those of the association.[30]

Most of the research that has helped document discrimination in health care has been conducted within medical school practice plans, not by outside critics or regulators. As suggested by Cowsert's clandestine battle with the Infirmary, racial disparities in referral patterns are a major contributor to disparities in outcomes. Borrowing directly from methods used in testing for housing and employment discrimination, 720 physicians at two national meetings for primary care physicians were given the same scenarios of a patient suffering from chest pain but varying the photos by race and sex of the purported patient. The physicians were significantly less likely to refer female and Black patients for cardiac catheterization.[31] It was not just the implicit biases of individual physician's referral decisions but the quality of the hospital where the patient was referred that contributed to the racial disparities in care. In an analysis of quality indicators on 123 hospitals for 320,970 adult patients, racial disparities in quality between hospitals rather than within hospitals accounted for most of the disparities.[32]

Some have demanded more help from organized medicine and the AAMC in ending racial bias.[33] Both spokespersons of the AMA and the AAMC have responded with outlines of strategic plans building on this literature and owning up to their past history of racial discrimination.[34]

The largest unanticipated organizational change since the implementation of Medicare and Medicaid was the emergence of medical school systems as dominant providers in most of the larger service areas. Most medical schools previously served as marginal providers of care, serving mostly the indigent in exchange for their use in teaching. In 1960 medical school revenue from their practice plans was less than 5 percent of the revenue they received from federal research funding.[35] By 2020 revenues for medical school practice plans and hospital services accounted for more than ninety-seven billion dollars and 63 percent of all medical school revenues.[36] Both in terms of their historical mission and greater dependence on government funding, they are more likely to share a compatible civil rights vision. The fears of a for-profit "new medical industrial complex" takeover of the delivery of health services never materialized.[37] Proprietary hospital chains served the more temporary health care equivalent of the expansion of private schools in the South, avoiding racial integration, cream skimming suburban private insurance patients but fading in relevance. Medical school systems now dominate most of the larger regional markets and continue to expand.

Voluntary initiatives do not take place in a vacuum. Money and laws shape them. The Title VI certification of hospitals for Medicare combined diverse voluntary initiatives with the money and laws to create remarkably effective programs. Voluntarism did not desegregate the hospitals even though there were plenty of people in leadership positions supportive of that goal. Providence Hospital tried to voluntarily desegregate, and they paid a price. Only the universal nature of the Medicare hospital payment program and the use of Title VI requirements made hospital desegregation possible.

The courts, however, have since rendered Title VI useless. In 2001 the Supreme Court delivered a devastating blow in *Alexander v. Sandoval* (532 US 275). The decision restricted the right of private parties to sue under Title VI only for "intentional" discrimination and left addressing discriminatory impact or "unintentional" discrimination to agency enforcement. Proving intentional discrimination is nearly impossible. Few are careless enough to provide concrete proof of bigotry. Critics argue that the Office for Civil Rights, responsible for such agency enforcement, has proved timid and ineffectual, fostering rather than combating discrimination.[38] Legislation has been proposed revising Title VI to again permit private civil suits for discriminatory "impact"(gross, unexplainable statistical disparities in treatment) and add suits for "negligence" (the failure to take adequate steps to monitor and correct discriminatory impacts).[39] Such a legislative revision, if nothing else, would give concerned and knowledgeable insiders more leverage to push for administrative and clinical reforms. In addition, the Affordable Care Act of 2010 (Section 1557) explicitly extends the Title VI prohibition against the use of federal funds to all providers of services, including physician practices and insurance plans. Physicians reimbursed under Part B of Medicare had originally been specifically exempted.

The ineffectiveness of Title VI, without legislative reforms, is painfully illustrated in the case of the last concerted attempt to use it to reduce inequities and segregation in care. A community advocacy group, Bronx REACH, investigated and lodged a civil rights complaint with the state attorney general against three major teaching centers in New York City (New York Presbyterian Hospital, the Mount Sinai Medical Center, and Montefiore Hospital). All three provided specialty outpatient care in two different settings—clinics and faculty practices. Testers, given a uniform script, called the hospital physician referral services to set up appointments for an endocrinologist (a physician specializing in disorders of the endocrine system such as diabetes) and a cardiologist. In both cases, as anticipated, all the uninsured and Medicaid patients, disproportionately Black and Hispanic, were referred to the clinic and the privately insured to the faculty practices. The care provided was not only separate but unequal. The faculty practice provided care by board certified specialists and after hour consultations with patients. The clinics had longer waiting times for appointments, did not provide any after hour management nor, as a matter policy, communicate or coordinate care with the patient's primary care physician. Bronx REACH's complaint claimed that these arrangements violated not just Title VI but Hill-Burton, New York State, and New York City requirements.[40]

The medical centers defended their practices as a "business necessity, dismissed REACH's proposal to combine the two practices in the same setting and began to sever legal ties between the private practice plans of faculty and the medical school to avoid any future challenges. Just as in the case of the Mobile Infirmary's medical staff, the New York City teaching hospitals could begin to claim that the faculty practices were independent operations for which they had no responsibility. The public officials, while acknowledging the validity of their complaint, indicated that there was nothing they could do. The last significant effort to use Title VI to end separate but unequal treatment ended. Only new legislation, as suggested earlier, can revive it as a tool.

The conditions that made it possible to effectively use Title VI in 1967 apply to the present ones.

1. **Timing:** The implementation of Medicare took place at the height of the civil rights movement. Similar rising demands for fundamental change exist now with the persistence of the COVID pandemic. Black Lives Matter demonstrations have swept the country, reinvigorating a civil rights movement fueled earlier by the Birmingham church bombing and the state trooper beating of marchers at the Pettus Bridge in Selma. The current timing is also opportune in terms of foreign conflicts. World War II did much to unite the country

in support of the Civil Rights agenda, but the Vietnam War destroyed that unity. The Ukrainian conflict appears close to uniting the country in support of democratic ideals as it was during World War II.

2. **Leaders:** A committed racially and economically diverse hidden team of collaborators captured the implementation of the Medicare program. That leadership team included minimum-wage hospital workers, local activists and eventually even President Lyndon Johnson. A similar consensus shapes concerns about disparities in outcomes and access to care for COVID and can push medical and public health reform well beyond it.

3. **Leverage:** Medicare's implementation was the first-time federal dollars were ever used to reshape the social purpose of private institutions. It worked in desegregating the nation's hospitals. Medicare funding made the difference in convincing hospital boards and management. That success soon led to prohibiting the use of federal funds in private institutions that discriminated based on sex. The leverage of public dollars can serve as a powerful force for change.

4. **Transparency:** It proved almost impossible to hide noncompliance in the Medicare effort to desegregate hospitals. However, the refusal of the Mobile Infirmary to share information on the racially selective referral patterns of its medical staff members shaped the battle over the Mobile Infirmary's Title VI certification. In the current age of electronic payment, referral patterns are far more transparent. Disparities in referral patterns that play a central role in current disparities can no longer be hidden.

Most disparities in treatment reflect larger social-economic conditions, not individual clinical decision-making biases of providers. Care is segregated because neighborhoods and insurance markets are segregated. Disparities in treatment reflect the disparities in providers available in poor versus affluent neighborhoods and in private versus Medicaid/uninsured markets. Dealing with bias and disparities involves dealing with social and not just clinical medicine. It is easier to do in larger more organized systems, such as regional medical school systems. It is also easier because everyone understands what needs to change. Only the will has been lacking but maybe that can change too. Structural discrimination should not be dismissed just as an excuse for doing nothing.

Residential segregation shapes health care segregation. Distance is by far the best predictor of where people seek care. Less segregated communities have better health statistics for all income levels, lower crime rates, and more intergenerational upward mobility. Low-income housing policies can reduce overall racial and economic segregation. Even some hospital systems have invested in such arrangements. More recent Black flight has followed white flight to the suburbs, suggesting an erosion of many of the older discriminatory barriers. Affordability (wealth and income inequalities) are the greatest deterrents to further reductions in segregation.

Wealth and income disparities, of course, also remain the biggest barriers to eliminating health disparities. Disparities in insurance coverage and payments to providers sort patients, contributing to existing gaps. If Medicaid payments matched private insurance payments, such sorting would be reduced. If hospital privileges, in the financial interest of hospitals, required physicians to accept all forms of insurance, that would also help. So would more universal comprehensive health insurance coverage. Plenty of interventions could reduce income inequalities—a higher minimum wage, expanded food and housing subsidies, tax rebates, etc. The array of options in narrowing the economic inequalities are only almost matched by the often-thoughtless arguments against them. I summarize three modest but persuasive ones:

Jack Geiger's Prescription: "At our first community health center, in the Mississippi Delta region—one of the poorest areas in the nation—people were drinking water from the drainage ditch. The insulation on these crumbling shacks was newspapers. Children were dying from the combination of infectious diarrhea and malnutrition. So, we intervened. We decided to start writing prescriptions for food. They would take the food order to the grocery store, which would bill the community health center, and we'd pay for it from the pharmacy budget. That led to this iconic exchange. The governor of Mississippi screamed at someone in the poverty program, who came down and screamed at me. 'What in God's name do you think you're doing giving away free food and charging it to the pharmacy? A pharmacy is for drugs to treat a disease.' And I said, 'The last time I looked at my textbooks, the most specific therapy for malnutrition was food.' And so, he went away because he couldn't think of anything to say to that."[41]

Impact of cash payments to low-income families on infant brain activity: A randomized clinical trial of 1,000 low-income mother-infant dyads was conducted. The high cash treatment group received $333 per month or a total of $4,000 during the first year of the infant's life. The low cash control group received $20 per month. EEG measured brain activity of the treatment group was higher than that of the control group. Giving monthly unconditional cash transfers to mothers experiencing poverty may change brain activity in their infants during the first year of life. Such patterns have been associated with the subsequent development of cognitive skills. A figure included in the report provided composite EKGs comparing the skulls of infants in the high and low cash groups. Warmer colors depicted greater brain activity. Even for a lay audience, the message was hard to miss. The paper received extensive press coverage.[42]

Investing in Infants and the Lasting Effects of Cash Transfers: The January 1 birth date cut off for income related child tax benefits provided the opportunity to match infants born in low-income families in December 1988 (the treatment group) and those born in January 1999 (the control group) and track their educational and early adult income outcomes through IRS, Census, and educational data sets. A thousand-dollar benefit in infancy translated into at least a 1–2 percent increase in earnings as a young adult, with earlier benefits showing up in higher math and reading scores and likelihood of high school graduation. During this critical window after birth persistent increases in family income distinguished the group receiving the tax benefit. Just the long-term increase in earnings of the infants in the treatment group as young adults more than paid for the tax benefit at birth through subsequent IRS tax revenues.[43]

Segregation and inequality of opportunities are root causes of injustice of all kinds. There is, in public investments, a "solidarity dividend" as so persuasively argued by Heather McGhee in *The Sum of Us*.[44] It beats paving over the pools in public parks as described in Chapter 5. It is a message capable of winning broad political support from conservatives concerned about efficiency and return on investment and activists concerned about social justice. It is a message that has long been embraced by many in medicine and public health. This approach was first advocated by nineteenth century medical pioneer Rudolph Virchow whose big idea was that "politics is nothing but medicine on a larger scale." It still resonates as it did in Geiger's iconic prescription in Mound Bayou.[45]

Much is riding on making the best of the current pressure for change. One could imagine Dr. Cowsert watching. Her life in the memories of the living and documents from the past have almost all disappeared. A couple of faded photos have been preserved. In one she is on a boat in fishing gear grinning. In the other she is well dressed in a pearl necklace at the service where she first professed her Catholic faith.

Only one document in her own handwriting has been saved. It is a "prescription" written for a friend, and nursing supervisor at Providence Hospital who was leaving for an assignment elsewhere. It became a keepsake saved by the friend for more than fifty years. May all of us have physicians that write such prescriptions and live lives as well reflected in that prescription as Dr. Cowsert.

> XXXXXX Rx for now
> To keep as sweet as you are
> To speak through your own deep belief and the
> way you live it the love of the
> God you so beautifully imitate
> To keep that little chin up and that smile show-
> ing often
> To remember how deeply loved you are and
> will be.
>
> 9/16/63 J. Cowsert, M.D.
> Refills PRN Times

NOTES

PREFACE

1. See, for example, Avedis Donabedian, *Exploring Quality Assessment and Monitoring: The Definition of Quality and Approaches to Its Assessment*, vol. 1 (Ann Arbor, MI: Health Administration Press, 1980).
2. David Barton Smith, *The Power to Heal: Civil Rights, Medicare, and the Struggle to Transform America's Health Care System* (Nashville, TN: Vanderbilt University Press, 2016).
3. Glenn Feldman, *The Disfranchisement Myth: Poor Whites and Suffrage Restriction in Alabama* (Athens: University of Georgia Press, 2004).
4. Amanda Gorman, *The Hill We Climb: An Inaugural Poem for the Country* (New York: Viking, 2021), 127, https://www.poetry.com/poem/60572/the-hill-we-climb.
5. Peter A. Hall, "Historical Institutionalism in Rationalist and Sociological Perspective," in *Explaining Institutional Change*, ed. James Mahoney and Kathleen Thelen (Cambridge: Cambridge University Press, 2010); Paul Pierson, "Path Dependence, Increasing Returns, and the Study of Politics," *Political Science Review* 33, no. 6/7 (2000): 251–67; Orfeo Fioretos, Tulia G. Falleti, and Adam Sheingate, *The Oxford Handbook of Historical Institutionalism* (Oxford: Oxford University Press, 2016).
6. Barack Obama, *A Promised Land* (New York: Crown, 2020), 421–22.
7. Clayborne Carson et al., *Reporting on Civil Rights: American Journalism 1941–1963* (New York: Library of America, 2003).

CHAPTER 1

1. Smith, *The Power to Heal*, 149–58.
2. Bernice Coreil, interview with author, Philadelphia, July 28, 2017, David Barton Smith Hospital Segregation Files, Charles L. Blockson Afro-American Collection, Temple University Libraries, Philadelphia, PA (hereafter Smith Hospital Segregation Files).
3. "Mobile Physician Fatally Wounded," *Mobile Register*, January 30, 1967.
4. Sister Mary Jane Code, telephone interview with author, Philadelphia, August 2019, Smith Hospital Segregation Files.
5. "Notes from Earl B. Wert Interview," May 6, 1998, Smith Hospital Segregation Files; John "Peet" Wert, telephone interview, Philadelphia, October 12, 2018, Smith Hospital Segregation Files.

6. John Wert, telephone interview, 2018, Smith Hospital Segregation Files.
7. "Mobile Physician Fatally Wounded," *Mobile Register*, January 30, 1967.
8. Code, telephone interview with author, 2019, Smith Hospital Segregation Files.

CHAPTER 2

1. See, for example, Richard Rothstein, *The Color of Law: A Forgotten History of How Our Government Segregated America* (New York: Liveright Publishing Corporation, 2017).
2. Even for schools, the *Brown* decision never resolved the issue. A "Southern Manifesto" pledging "massive resistance" signed by almost all federal legislators from the South lives on. It has more recently surfaced as a battle over passing state laws banning the teaching of "critical race theory" and making it a crime to teach anything about transgender identity in a public classroom. According to some, the longer-range conservative agenda is to eliminate public school altogether. Most citizens support public schools, which they still have, just as they support some version of a Medicare-for-all public insurance program, which they don't. They also support requiring school attendance to a certain age to avoid child labor abuses and assuring that all citizens would have the skills to participate effectively in a democracy. Ironically, this was part of the Progressive agenda more than a century ago. Jill Lepore, "The Parent Trap," *New Yorker*, March 21, 2022.
3. Mattie Gadson, taped interview with author, April 17, 1996, Smith Hospital Segregation Files.
4. David W. Southern, *The Malignant Heritage: Yankee Progressives and the Negro Question, 1901–1914* (Chicago: Loyola University Press, 1968), 10–17.
5. David L. Lewis, *W. E. B. Du Bois: A Biography* (New York: Holt Paperbacks, 2009).
6. Equal Justice Initiative, "Lynching in America: Confronting the Legacy of Racial Terror, Third Edition" (Montgomery, AL, 2017), https://eji.org/reports/lynching-in-america.
7. Steven J. Jager, "Dyer Anti-Lynching Bill (1922)," Black Past, August 19, 2012, https://www.blackpast.org/african-american-history/dyer-anti-lynching-bill-1922.
8. David Zucchino, *Wilmington's Lie: The Murderous Coup of 1898 and the Rise of White Supremacy* (New York: Atlantic Monthly Press, 2020).
9. Brent Staples, "The Burning of Black Wall Street, Revisited," *New York Times*, June 19, 2020, https://www.nytimes.com/2020/06/19/opinion/tulsa-race-riot-massacre-graves.html; Karlos K. Hill, *Tulsa, 1921: Reporting a Massacre* (Norman: University of Oklahoma Press, 2019).
10. Community efforts to provide a full accounting in Tulsa began in anticipation of the centennial of the massacre in 2021. The outbreak of the COVID pandemic in 2020 delayed exhuming the bodies in a long concealed common grave. But President Trump was not delayed. He launched his first public reelection campaign rally in Tulsa on June 20, 2020. Professing no awareness of the symbolic message of such an act, Trump followed in the footsteps of other politicians claiming similar innocence in sending racist "dog whistles" to their base. Ronald Reagan, for example, launched his first presidential campaign rally at the Nashoba County,

Mississippi Fair on August 3, 1980. Reagan spoke for a return to the supremacy of state rights a few miles away from the earthen dam where the bodies of civil rights voter registration workers Chaney, Goodman, and Schwerner had been buried sixteen years earlier by the Klan. In Tulsa, the current mayor, concerned with the impact any kind of reparations for the families of victims would have on property taxes, might well prefer that the unmarked mass graves just be left that way. Caleb Gayle, "100 Years after the Tulsa Massacre, What Does Justice Look Like?" *New York Times Magazine*, May 25, 2021, https://www.nytimes.com/2021/05/25/ magazine/tulsa-race-massacre-1921-greenwood.html.

11. Roberta Senechal de la Roche, *In Lincoln's Shadow: The 1908 Race Riot in Springfield, Illinois* (Carbondale: Southern Illinois University Press, 2008).

12. "Founding and Early Years," *NAACP: A Century in the Fight for Freedom*, Library of Congress, Exhibitions, 2021, https://www.loc.gov/exhibits/naacp/founding-and-early-years.html.

13. C. Vann Woodward, *The Strange Career of Jim Crow* (New York: Oxford University Press, 1955).

14. Robert Lewis Stevenson, *The Strange Case of Dr. Jekyll and Mr. Hyde* (London: Longmans, Green and Company, 1886).

15. Southern, *The Malignant Heritage*, 54.

16. Sarah Bahr, "Roosevelt Statue to Head to Presidential Library in North Dakota," *New York Times*, November 19, 2021, https://www.nytimes.com/2021/11/19/arts/design/roosevelt-statue-north-dakota.html.

17. Peter M. Ascoli, *Julius Rosenwald: The Man Who Built Sears, Roebuck and Advanced the Cause of Black Education in the American South* (Bloomington: Indiana University Press, 2006).

18. Hasia R. Diner, *Julius Rosenwald: Repairing the World* (New Haven, CT: Yale University Press, 2017).

19. David Barton Smith, *Health Care Divided: Race and Healing a Nation* (Ann Arbor: University of Michigan Press, 1999), 79–80.

20. Greensboro interview with Cong. L. Richardson Preyer, June 28, 1996, Smith Hospital Segregation Files.

21. Quoted in Stefan Kühl, *The Nazi Connection: Eugenics, American Racism, and German National Socialism* (New York: Oxford University Press, 2002), 13.

22. Quoted in Kühl, *The Nazi Connection*, 16.

23. Kühl, *The Nazi Connection*.

24. Isabel Wilkerson, *Caste: The Origins of Our Discontents* (New York: Random House, 2020).

25. Stephen Skowronek, "The Reassociation of Ideas and Purposes: Racism, Liberalism, and the American Political Tradition," *American Political Science Review* 100, no. 3 (August 2006): 385–401.

26. Woodrow Wilson, *A History of the American People* (Harper & Brothers, 1917).

27. Wilson, *A History of the American People*, 60–62.

28. Eric S. Yellin, *Racism in the Nation's Service: Government Workers and the Color Line in Woodrow Wilson's America* (Chapel Hill: University of North Carolina Press, 2013).

29. "Mr. Trotter and Mr. Wilson," *Crisis* 9 (January 1915): 119–20.

30. Yellin, *Racism in the Nation's Service*, 164.

31. Samuel Walker, *Presidents and Civil Liberties from Wilson to Obama: A Story of Poor Custodians* (New York: Cambridge University Press, 2012).

32. Wilson, *A History of the American People.*

33. Abraham Lincoln, "Gettysburg Address," November 19, 1863, American Battlefield Trust, accessed June 26, 2023, https://www.battlefields.org/learn/primary-sources/abraham-lincolns-gettysburg-address.

34. Anne Hollmuller, "The Dedication of the Lincoln Memorial," *Boundary Stones Blog* (Washington, DC: WETA, 2018), https://boundarystones.weta.org/2018/04/18/dedication-lincoln-memorial.

35. Kendrick A. Clements, *The Presidency of Woodrow Wilson* (Lawrence: University Press of Kansas, 1992), ix.

36. Brett Tomlinson and Carlett Spike, "Princeton Renames Wilson School and Residential College, Citing Former President's Racism," *Princeton Alumni Weekly,* June 27, 2020, https://paw.princeton.edu/print/232221.

37. It is more complicated and hopelessly intertwined with racism, as well documented in Jesse Tarbert's recent book, *When Good Government Meant Big Government: The Quest to Expand Federal Power, 1913–1933* (New York: Columbia University Press, 2022). The two national parties turned themselves inside out over the proper role of the national government, reflecting the shifting influence of the Southern view of white supremacy on both.

38. John M. Barry, *The Great Influenza: The Story of the Deadliest Pandemic in History* (New York: Random House, 2018), 197–227.

39. Barry, *The Great Influenza,* 204.

40. Barry, *The Great Influenza,* 220–24.

41. Frank Fitzpatrick, "Dining Room of Dead Bodies," *Philadelphia Inquirer,* April 28, 2020.

42. Barry, *The Great Influenza,* 505.

43. The Espionage Act of 1917 and the eventual creation of the FBI to help enforce it was used to curtail left-leaning opposition to the war and then to attempt to control civil rights activism. The Act resurfaced as a justification for efforts to prevent leaks in top-secret documents for the Department of Justice and FBI raid of former President Trump's residence in 2022.

44. In a final irony, Wilson succumbed to the pandemic in much the same way President Trump did. He failed to achieve his dream—a peace assuring that World War I would indeed be the "war to end all wars." That accomplishment, despite his racial views, would have kept him in the top ranks of US presidents. Yet that failure may be the fault of the influenza pandemic of 1918. Wilson arrived in Paris in 1919 to negotiate the peace treaty during an influenza upsurge. Wilson's closest confidant Edward House, his daughter Margaret, his wife's secretary, and Dr. Cary Grayson, his personal physician and advisor, all had been infected. Even Britain's Lloyd George and France's Clemenceau, the other key parties to the peace negotiations, had been infected. As these negotiations dragged on, Wilson continued to insist on a peace without the winners just dividing up the spoils. On April 3, however, Wilson became violently ill with a fever of 103, coughing, and diarrhea. For several days Wilson lay in his bed unable to move. His aides noticed a profound change in mental capacities. He was never the same again.

The condition, as diagnosed by Dr. Grayson and as verified by John Barry in his carefully documented assessment in *The Great Influenza,* was not the result of a minor stroke as some historians concluded, but a result of influenza (387). In his case, it lingered, affecting his physical stamina and mental concentration. The stroke that would later incapacitate him may also have been a consequence of the influenza infection. In any event, he abandoned his previous positions and yielded to everything Clemenceau had demanded. This included reparations from Germany, which would now be required to accept full responsibility for the war, ceding territory and colonies to its adversaries. Wilson also conceded to Italy much of its demands for expanded territory from Germany and agreed to Japan's insistence that it take over German concessions in China. Wilson had once insisted that lasting peace could only be achieved by "a peace without victory." The conditions imposed on Germany produced economic hardship, a nationalistic reaction, and political chaos that contributed to the rise of Adolf Hitler. The agreement appalled many of Wilson's key diplomatic advisers, three of whom resigned. One, Adolf Berle, who later became Secretary of State, wrote Wilson, "you had so little faith in the millions of men, like me in every nation who had faith in you. Our government has consented now to deliver the suffering peoples of the world to new oppressions, subjections and dismemberments—a new century of war" (Barry, *The Great Influenza,* 388). Four months later Wilson suffered a major debilitating stroke probably caused by brain hemorrhages, a complication often resulting from the virus. He would serve out his term incapacitated with his wife and his personal physician acting as surrogates. The influenza pandemic of 1918 may have ended one war but produced another century of them.

45. National Center for Health Statistics, "Leading Causes of Death, 1900–1998," CDC, accessed July 8, 2023, https://www.cdc.gov/nchs/data/dvs/lead1900_98.pdf.

46. "Health in the United States 2019, Table 5," Centers for Disease Control and Prevention National Center for Health Statistics, 2021, https://www.cdc.gov/nchs/data/hus/2019/005-508.pdf.

47. "Health in the United States 2019, Table 5."

48. Centers for Disease Control and Prevention, "NCHS—Infant Mortality Rates by Race: United States, 1915–2013," June 5, 2020, https://data.cdc.gov/NCHS/NCHS-Infant-Mortality-Rates-by-Race-United-States-/ddsk-zebd; National Center for Health Statistics, *Health, United States 2010* (Hyattsville, MD: Department of Health and Human Services, 2011).

49. Matthew J. Best et al., "Racial Disparities in the Use of Surgical Procedures in the US," *JAMA Surgery,* 2021, E1–E9. The surgical rate disparities used in this evaluation included angioplasty, spinal fusion, coronary artery bypass grafting, carotid endarterectomy, total hip arthroplasty, total knee arthroplasty, valve replacement, appendectomy, and colorectal resection.

50. Peter J. Hotez, *Preventing the Next Pandemic: Vaccine Diplomacy in a Time of Anti-science* (Baltimore: Johns Hopkins University Press, 2021).

51. Anne Case and Angus Deaton, *Deaths of Despair and the Future of Capitalism* (Princeton, NJ: Princeton University Press, 2020).

52. Frank M. Snowden, *Epidemics and Society: From the Black Death to the Present* (New Haven, CT: Yale University Press, 2020).

53. Ronald Hamowy, "The Early Development of Medical Licensing Laws in the United States, 1875–1900," *Journal of Libertarian Studies* 3, no. 1 (1979): 73.

54. Hamowy, "The Early Development," 77.

55. Hamowy, "The Early Development," 77.

56. Hamowy, "The Early Development," 77.

57. Harriet J. Scarupa, "W. Montague Cobb: His Long, Storied, Battle-Scarred Life," *New Directions* 5, no. 2 (1988), https://dh.howard.edu/newdirections/vol15/iss2/2.

58. Black hearses also served in the search for justice as well as for hospital accommodations. A borrowed hearse transported Thurgood Marshall and his legal team from Charlotte to the US District Court in the *Briggs v. Elliot*, 342 US 350 (1952) school desegregation case in Summerton, South Carolina. It was the first of five cases that would be combined into the *Brown v. Board of Education* Supreme Court decision. Facing threats on their lives, they traveled at night from Charlotte, sitting out of sight on the floor in the back of the hearse. According to Reginald Hawkins, DDS, a civil rights activist in Charlotte who made the arrangements, Marshall shared his good bourbon and off-color jokes with the other passengers. The leader of the school desegregation effort in Summerton survived a drive-by shooting. All those who participated in bringing the case were fired from their jobs and all, including the judge who voted supporting their case, left the state soon afterward. Their courage would be honored in South Carolina a half-century later after most of them were dead. Taped interview with Reginald Hawkins, Philadelphia, PA, 2000, Smith Hospital Segregation Files.

59. Alfred Maund, "The Untouchables: The Meaning of Segregation in Hospitals," 1952, Library of Social and Economic Aspects of Medicine of Michael M. Davis, The Drs. Barry and Bobbi Coller Rare Book Room, New York Academy of Medicine Library, New York City.

60. Quentin Young, taped interview with author, Philadelphia, June 14, 1997, Smith Hospital Segregation Files.

61. Frederick C. Waite, "Grave Robbing in New England," *Bulletin of the Medical Library Association* 33, no. 3 (July 1945): 272–94.

62. W. Montague Cobb, "Surgery and the Negro Physician: Some Parallels in Background," *Journal of the National Medical Association* 43 (1951): 148.

63. Loyal Davis, *Fellowship of Surgeons: A History of the American College of Surgeons* (Chicago: American College of Surgeons, 1960), https://archive.org/details/FellowshipOfSurgeons.

64. Davis, *Fellowship of Surgeons.*

65. David L. Nahrwold and Peter J. Kernahan, *A Century of Surgeons and Surgery* (Chicago: American College of Surgeons, 2012): 34.

66. Vanessa Northington Gamble, *Making a Place for Ourselves* (New York: Oxford University Press, 1995), 70–104.

67. Abraham Flexner, *Medical Education in the United States and Canada: A Report to the Carnegie Foundation for the Advancement of Teaching* (New York: Carnegie Foundation for the Advancement of Teaching, 1910).

68. Andrew H. Beck, "The Flexner Report and the Standardization of American Medical Education," *JAMA* 291, no. 17 (2004): 2139–40.

69. Flexner, *Medical Education,* 136.

70. Flexner, *Medical Education*, 181.
71. H. S. Berliner, "A Larger Perspective on the Flexner Report," *International Journal of Health Services: Planning, Administration, Evaluation* 5, no. 4 (1975): 590, https://doi.org/10.2190/F31Q-592N-056K-VETL.
72. Flexner, *Medical Education*, 180.
73. Flexner, *Medical Education*, 180.
74. James H. Jones, *Bad Blood: The Tuskegee Syphilis Experiment* (New York: Free Press, 1981).
75. Rebecca Skloot, *The Immortal Life of Henrietta Lacks* (New York: Random House, 2011).
76. Thomas P. Duffy, "The Flexner Report—100 Years Later," *Yale Journal of Biology and Medicine* 84, no. 3 (September 2011): 269–76.
77. Gabrielle Redford, "AAMC Renames Prestigious Abraham Flexner Award in Light of Racist and Sexist Writings," Association of American Medical Colleges, Nov. 17, 2020, https://www.aamc.org/news-insights/aamc-renames-prestigious-abraham-flexner-award-light-racist-and-sexist-writings.
78. For a fascinating account see Richard D. deShazo, ed., *The Racial Divide in American Medicine: Black Physicians and the Struggle for Justice in Health Care* (Jackson: University Press of Mississippi, 2018), 71–82.

CHAPTER 3

1. World Health Organization, "Universal Health Coverage," accessed May 25, 2023, https://www.who.int/news-room/fact-sheets/detail/universal-health-coverage-(uhc).
2. Deborah Stone, "The Struggle for the Soul of Health Insurance," *Journal of Health Politics, Policy and Law* 18, no. 2 (1993): 287–317.
3. Frederick L. Hoffman, "Race Traits and Tendencies of the American Negro," *American Economic Association* 1, no. 1–3 (1896): 1–329.
4. The history of life and health insurance for Black people is rich in ironies. As enslaved persons, they were the first in the United States to have their lives protected. That protection prevented owners from losing money from their death. Slave owners could contract their "property" out for risky work such as in mines. Northern-based firms such as what became Chase Manhattan, Aetna, and New York Life are now in the process of making amends for their role in insuring the lives of enslaved persons. As freed persons, however, Black policy holders were the last to be served by private life and health insurance. Such discrimination based on race opened an opportunity for Black entrepreneurs. More than forty-three Black-owned life insurance companies were established. Some of their founders were among the nation's first Black millionaires. Many Black owners of life insurance companies were also leaders in the subsequent civil rights struggles. Discriminatory pricing of life insurance policies for Black Americans did not end until the 1950s. Settlement of all the historical race-based pricing of life insurance policies didn't take place until the first decade of the twenty-first century. Mary L. Heen, "Ending Jim Crow Life Insurance Rates," *Northwestern Journal of Law and Social Policy* 4, no. 2 (Fall 2009): 360–99.

5. Robert I. Field, *The Mother of Invention: How the Government Created "Free Market" Health Care* (New York: Oxford University Press, 2014).

6. Eric C. Schneider et al., "Mirror, Mirror 2021—Reflecting Poorly: Health Care in the U.S. Compared to Other High-Income Countries" (New York: The Commonwealth Fund, August 2021), https://www.commonwealthfund.org/publications/fund-reports/2021/aug/mirror-mirror-2021-reflecting-poorly. The ten countries compared to the US are Australia, Canada, France, Germany, the Netherlands, New Zealand, Norway, Sweden, Switzerland, and the United Kingdom.

7. Nicholas Laham, *Why the United States Lacks a National Health Insurance Program* (Westport, CT: Greenwood Press, 1993); Colin Gordon, *Dead on Arrival: The Politics of Health Care in Twentieth-Century America* (Princeton, NJ: Princeton University Press, 2004).

8. Jill Quadagno, *The Color of Welfare: How Racism Undermined the War on Poverty* (Oxford: Oxford University Press, 1994).

9. Angie Maxwell and Todd Shields, *The Long Southern Strategy: How Chasing White Voters in the South Changed American Politics* (New York: Oxford University Press, 2019).

10. Smith, *The Power to Heal*, 139.

11. Smith, *The Power to Heal*, 168–69.

12. David T. Beito, "The 'Lodge Practice Evil' Reconsidered: Medical Care through Fraternal Societies, 1900-1930," *Journal of Urban History* 23, no. 5 (1997): 569–600.

13. John Hatch, taped interview with author, Philadelphia, August 29, 1996, Smith Hospital Segregation Files.

14. Paul Starr, *The Social Transformation of American Medicine* (New York: Harper Collins, 1982), 151.

15. Monte M. Poen, *Harry S. Truman versus the Medical Lobby* (Columbia: University of Missouri Press, 1979), 151.

16. Poen, *Harry S. Truman*, 145.

17. See, for example, David Barton Smith, "The Politics of Racial Disparities: Desegregating the Hospitals in Jackson, Mississippi," *Milbank Quarterly* 83, no. 5 (2005): 247–69.

18. See, for example, Ronald Numbers, *Almost Persuaded: American Physicians and Compulsory Health Insurance, 1912–1920* (Baltimore, MD: Johns Hopkins Press, 1978); Paul Starr, *The Social Transformation of American Medicine* (New York: Harper Collins, 1982); Roy Lubove, *The Struggle for Social Security, 1900–1935* (Cambridge, MA: Harvard University Press, 1968); Monte M. Poen, *Harry S. Truman*; Alan B. Cohen et al., eds., *Medicare and Medicaid at 50* (New York, 2015); Beatrix Hoffman, *Health Care for Some: Rights and Rationing in the United States since 1930* (Chicago: The University of Chicago Press, 2012).

19. David Barton Smith, "Jim Crow Medicine and the Elusive Pursuit of Universal Care," in *The Oxford Handbook of American Medical History*, edited by James A. Schafer Jr., Richard M. Mizelle, and Helen K. Valier (New York: Oxford University Press, in press).

20. Southern white voters sided overwhelmingly for Wilson anyway. With the

Republican party split in two through the creation of the Progressive Party, Wilson won by a landslide. Racial politics would continue to block action on health insurance.

21. Numbers, *Almost Persuaded.*

22. Isidore Sydney Falk, Margaret Klem, and Nathan Sinai, "The Incidence of Illness and the Receipt and Costs of Medical Care among Representative Families," Publications of the Committee on the Cost of Medical Care, no. 26. (Chicago: University of Chicago Press, 1932), 51.

23. "The Committee on the Cost of Medical Care," *JAMA* 99, no. 23 (1932): 1950–52.

24. "Socialized Medicine Is Urged in Survey," *New York Times*, November 30, 1932.

25. Arthur J. Altmeyer, *The Formative Years of Social Security* (Madison: University of Wisconsin Press, 1966), 27.

26. Harry S. Truman, "Special Message to Congress Recommending a Comprehensive Health Program," in *Public Papers of the Presidents of the United States: Harry S. Truman, 1945–1953* (Washington, DC: US Government Printing Office, 1966).

27. One of the profound ironies of this rapid transformation is that the same voluntary ownership patterns that had insulated hospitals from desegregation now expedited it. A voluntary hospital board member's primary responsibility is a fiduciary one to protect its charitable assets. Once it was clear that failure to comply with Title VI requirements would bankrupt a facility and that compliance would result in windfall opportunities for expansion, few had difficulty making the right decision. Desegregation was implemented quietly, even secretly, without any notification to the community. This rollout offered no opportunities for protests or delayed implementation. The other profound irony was that there was nothing voluntary about it. It was a universal requirement. No hospital could remain segregated and expect to cater to those who preferred segregated services. For those who wanted Medicare reimbursement for their care or Medicare payment for the services they received, there was no "freedom of choice."

28. Smith, *Health Care Divided*, 200–211.

29. Nancy Krieger et al., "The Fall and Rise of US Inequities in Premature Mortality 1960-2002," *PLOS Medicine* 5, no. 2 (February 2008): e46.

30. Jonathan Oberlander and Theodore R. Marmor, "The Road Not Taken: What Happened to Medicare for All?," in *Medicare and Medicaid at 50: America's Entitlement Programs in the Age of Affordable Care*, ed. Alan B. Cohen et al. (New York: Oxford University Press, 2015), 55–74.

31. See, for example, Karen E. Joynt, E. John Orav, and Ashish K. Jha, "Thirty-Day Readmission Rates for Medicare Beneficiaries by Race and Site of Care," *JAMA* 305, no. 7 (February 16, 2011): 475–681.

32. Roosa Tikkanen, "Multinational Comparisons of Health Systems Data" (New York: Commonwealth Fund, August 29, 2018), https://doi.org/10.26099/y2kb-sx06.

33. David Barton Smith et al., "Separate and Unequal: Racial Segregation and Disparities in Quality across U.S. Nursing Homes," *Health Affairs* 26, no. 5 (2007): 1448–58; David B. Smith et al., "Racial Disparities in Access to Long-Term Care: The Illusive Pursuit of Equity," *Journal of Health Politics, Policy and Law* 33, no. 5 (2008): 861–81.

34. David Barton Smith, "Population Ecology and the Racial Integration of Hospitals and Nursing Homes in the United States," *Milbank Quarterly* 68, no. 4 (1990): 561–96; David Barton Smith, "Addressing Racial Inequities in Health Care: Civil Rights Monitoring and Report Cards," *Journal of Health Politics, Policy and Law* 23, no. 1 (1998): 75–107.

35. Richard M. Nixon, "Special Message to the Congress Proposing a National Health Strategy," American Presidency Project, UC Santa Barbara, February 18, 1971, https://www.presidency.ucsb.edu/documents/special-message-the-congress-proposing-national-health-strategy.

36. Ronald Reagan, "Inaugural Address 1981," Ronald Reagan Presidential Library and Museum, January 20, 1981, https://www.reaganlibrary.gov/archives/speech/inaugural-address-1981.

37. Stuart M. Butler, "Assuring Affordable Health Care for All Americans," The Heritage Lectures (Washington, DC: The Heritage Foundation, 1989), https://www.heritage.org/social-security/report/assuring-affordable-health-care-all-americans.

38. Mark V. Pauly et al., "A Plan for 'Responsible National Health Insurance,'" *Health Affairs* 10, no. 1 (January 1991): 5–25, https://doi.org/10.1377/hlthaff.10.1.5.

39. Avik Roy, "The Tortuous History of Conservatives and the Individual Mandate," *Forbes*, February 7, 2012.

40. The Cato Institute, "Universal Health Care" (Cato Institute, 2018), https://web.archive.org/web/20180216175537/https://www.cato.org/research/universal-health-care.

41. Daniel Villarreal, "69 Percent of Americans Want Medicare for All, Including 46 Percent of Republicans, New Poll Says," *Newsweek*, 2020), https://www.newsweek.com/69-percent-americans-want-medicare-all-including-46-percent-republicans-new-poll-says-1500187.

CHAPTER 4

1. "America's Most Endangered Rivers for 2017: Mobile Bay Basin [AL]," American Rivers, July 6, 2017, https://web.archive.org/web/20170706051120/https://www.americanrivers.org/endangered-rivers/mobile-bay-basin-al.

2. Jay Higginbotham, "Discovery, Exploration, and Colonization of Mobile to 1711," in *Mobile: The New History of Alabama's First City*, ed. Michael V. R. Thomason (Tuscaloosa: University of Alabama Press, 2001).

3. Higginbotham, "Discovery, Exploration," 16.

4. Alexander Koch et al., "Earth System Impacts of the European Arrival and Great Dying in the Americas after 1492," *Quaternary Science Reviews* 207 (March 1, 2019): 13–36, https://doi.org/10.1016/j.quascirev.2018.12.004.

5. Wyatte Grantham-Philips, "On the Navajo Nation, COVID-19 Death Toll Is Higher than Any US State: Here's How You Can Support Community Relief," *USA TODAY*, October 24, 2020.

6. Ronald Segal, *The Black Diaspora: Five Centuries of the Black Experience Outside Africa* (New York: Farrar, Straus and Giroux, 1995).

7. Michael B. A. Oldstone, *Viruses, Plagues, and History* (New York: Oxford University Press, 2020).

8. Sven Beckert and Seth Rockman, *Slavery's Capitalism: A New History of American Economic Development* (Philadelphia: University of Pennsylvania Press, 2016), 2.
9. Beckert and Rockman, 15.
10. Craig Steven Wilder, *Ebony and Ivy: Race, Slavery, and the Troubled History of America's Universities* (New York: Bloomsbury Publishing USA, 2013).
11. Rachel L. Swarns, "272 Slaves Were Sold to Save Georgetown. What Does It Owe Its Descendants?," *New York Times*, April 16, 2016, www.nytimes.com/2016/04/17/us/georgetown-university-search-for-slave-descendents.html.
12. Harriet E. Amos Doss, "Cotton City, 1813–1860," in Thomason, *Mobile*, 79.
13. Natalie S. Robertson, *The Slave Ship* Clotilda *and the Making of AfricaTown, USA* (Westport, CT: Praeger, 2008).
14. Zora Neale Hurston, *Barracoon: The Story of the Last "Black Cargo"* (New York: Amistad, 2018).
15. James P. Delgado et al. Clotilda: *The History and Archaeology of the Last Slave Ship* (Tuscaloosa: University of Alabama Press, 2023).
16. Samuel L. Williamson and Louis P. Cain, "Measuring Slavery in 2020 Dollars," Measuring Worth, 2023. https://www.measuringworth.com/slavery.php.
17. Beckert and Rockman, *Slavery's Capitalism*; Matthew Desmond, "Capitalism," in *The 1619 Project*, ed. Nikole Hannah-Jones (New York: One World, 2021), 165–85.
18. Caitlin Rosenthal, "Slavery's Scientific Management: Masters and Managers," in *Slavery's Capitalism*, ed. Sven Beckert and Seth Rockman (Philadelphia: University of Pennsylvania Press, 2016), 62–86.
19. Rachel L. Swarns, "Insurance Policies on Slaves: New York Life's Complicated Past," December 18, 2016, http://www.nytimes.com/2016/12/18/us/insurance-policies-on-slaves-new-york-lifes-complicated-past.html.
20. Harriet E. Amos Doss, "Cotton City, 1813–1860," in Thomason, *Mobile*.
21. Doss, "Cotton City," 75.
22. William Warren Rogers et al., *Alabama: The History of a Deep South State* (Tuscaloosa: University of Alabama Press, 1994), 111.
23. Rogers et al., *Alabama*, 111.
24. Rogers et al., *Alabama*, 111.
25. Rogers et al., *Alabama*, 110.
26. Rogers et al., *Alabama*, 197.
27. "The Battle of Shiloh, 1862," Eyewitness to History, 2004, http://www.eyewitnesstohistory.com/pfshiloh.htm.
28. "The Battle of Shiloh."
29. Emily S. Renschler and Janet Monge, "The Samuel George Morton Cranial Collection," *Expedition* 50, no. 3 (2008): 34.
30. Stephan Salisbury, "Origins of Skulls Held by Penn Hard to Untangle," *Philadelphia Inquirer*, February 16, 2021.
31. The collection of skulls also includes ones of Black Philadelphia residents "harvested" by Morton from the potter's field adjacent to Philadelphia General Hospital in West Philadelphia. About half the occupants were Black, many of them slaves. They were stacked on top of each other in pits twenty feet deep. Paul Wolff Mitchell, "Black Philadelphians in the Samuel George Morton Cranial Collection." Accessed April 26, 2022. The depression created by the site was later

filled in 1895 by Franklin Field, the university's football stadium. The contents of the potter's field remain buried beneath the football stadium. Morton's skull collection remained on open display in a classroom just across the street in the university's museum until 2020. Anger over this collection by Black neighbors increased with revelations that the Museum had included in a recent display the bones of a child killed in the Philadelphia Police firebombing of the home of a member of Black militant group MOVE in West Philadelphia in 1985. Abdul-Aliy Muhammad, "Laying Questions to Rest: Treatment of MOVE Remains Demands Probe," *Philadelphia Inquirer*, May 9, 2021.

32. C. Loring Brace, "The 'Ethnology' of Josiah Clark Nott," *Bulletin of the New York Academy of Medicine* 504 (April 1974): 524.

33. Henry M. McKiven, "Secession, War, and Reconstruction, 1850–1874," in Thomason, *Mobile*, 102.

34. McKiven, "Secession," 104–105.

35. McKiven, "Secession," 107.

36. McKiven, "Secession," 106–7.

37. McKiven, "Secession," 107.

38. Paul Brueske, *The Last Siege: The Mobile Campaign, Alabama 1865* (Philadelphia: Casemate, 2018), 139.

39. Equal Justice Initiative, *Reconstruction in America: Racial Violence after the Civil War: 1865–1876* (Montgomery, AL: Equal Justice Initiative, 2020), 50.

40. Erin Blakemore, "President Andrew Johnson Was Impeached for Firing a Cabinet Officer," History.com, 2019, https://www.history.com/news/ andrew-johnson-impeachment-tenure-of-office-act.

41. Alabama Constitutional Convention, "Alabama State Constitution, 1865," Article IV, Section 36, https://www.wethepeoplealabama.org/_files/ugd/ e493c1_3e4a52785ef0415387f4dd6b5a885364.pdf.

42. Douglas A. Blackmon, *Slavery by Another Name: The Re-Enslavement of Black Americans from the Civil War to World War II* (New York: Anchor Books, 2008).

43. "Incarceration Rates by Country 2023," World Population Review, accessed July 8, 2023, https://worldpopulationreview.com/country-rankings/ incarceration-rates-by-country.

44. McKiven, "Secession," 115.

45. Michelle Alexander, *The New Jim Crow: Mass Incarceration in the Age of Colorblindness* (New York: The New Press, 2010).

46. Rogers et al., *Alabama*, 243.

47. McKiven, "Secession," 117.

48. McKiven, "Secession," 116–17.

49. McKiven, "Secession," 119.

50. Quoted in McKiven, "Secession," 124.

51. Quoted in McKiven, "Secession," 125–125.

52. Quoted in McKiven, "Secession," 114.

53. John David Smith and J. Vincent Lowery, eds., *The Dunning School* (Lexington: University Press of Kentucky, 2013), 1.

54. W. E. B. Du Bois, *Black Reconstruction in America* (New York: Harcourt Brace, 1935).

55. Christopher MacGregor Scribner, "Progress versus Tradition in Mobile, 1900–1920," in Thomason, *Mobile*, 168–69.

CHAPTER 5

1. John B. Knox, "Opening Remarks 1901 Proceedings of the Constitutional Convention, Day 2 of 54, Page 8," 1901. http://www.legislature.state.al.us/aliswww/history/constitutions/1901/proceedings/1901_proceedings_vol1/day2.html.

2. Glenn Feldman, *The Disfranchisement Myth: Poor Whites and Suffrage Restriction in Alabama* (Athens: University of Georgia Press, 2004).

3. Campbell Robertson, "Alabama Simmers Before Vote on Its Constitution's Racist Language," *New York Times*, October 31, 2012, https://www.nytimes.com/2012/10/31/us/alabama-simmers-before-vote-on-its-constitutions-racist-language.html.

4. Institute on Taxation and Economic Policy, "Who Pays? A Distributional Analysis of the Tax Systems of All 50 States, 6th Edition," 2018, https://itep.sfo2.digitaloceanspaces.com/itep-whopays-Alabama.pdf; World Population Review, "Per Pupil Spending by State 2021," 2021, https://worldpopulationreview.com/state-rankings/per-pupil-spending-by-state.

5. "Alabama Constitution of 1901," Wikipedia, last edited June 14, 2023, at 20:39 (UTC), https://en.wikipedia.org/wiki/Alabama_Constitution_of_1901.

6. Brian Lyman, "Alabama Constitution Committee Approves Plan to Remove Racist Language," *Montgomery Advertiser*, November 3, 2021, https://www.montgomeryadvertiser.com/story/news/2021/11/03/alabama-constitution-committee-approves-plan-remove-racist-language/6244819001.

7. Fair Ballot Commission, "Ballot Statement for the Constitution of Alabama of 2022," Alabama Secretary of State, https://www.sos.alabama.gov/sites/default/files/election-2022/BallotStatementForConstitutionofAlabamaof2022.pdf

8. Rogers et al., *Alabama*, 352.

9. One of the reasons to justify the Constitution's passage was to end the fraud perpetrated by white Democratic leaders in the Black Belt counties, with their concentration of cotton farming and the state's Black population. These leaders had a tradition of stuffing the ballot boxes with Black votes to their liking to assure control of the state. Statewide the reported vote on ratification of the Constitution was 108,613 in favor and 81,734 opposed. The vote in the Black Belt counties was 36,224 in favor and 5,471 opposed, and the vote in the other counties was 76,236 opposed and 72,389 in favor. (The vote in Mobile County was even more strongly opposed to ratification). It is unlikely that almost every eligible Black voter in those counties voted to support their own disenfranchisement. Rogers et al., *Alabama*, 353.

10. "The Citizens of Alabama Declare for White Supremacy," *Montgomery Advertiser*, November 12, 1901.

11. Keith Nicholls, "Politics and Civil Rights in Post-World War II Mobile," in Thomason, *Mobile*, 271.

12. Michael W. Fitzgerald, *Urban Emancipation: Popular Politics in Reconstruction Mobile, 1860-1890* (Baton Rouge: Louisiana State University Press, 2002), 266–67.

13. David Ernest Alsobrook, "Alabama's Port City: Mobile during the Progressive Era, 1896–1917," PhD diss., (Auburn University, 1983).

14. Fredrick Douglas Richardson, *The Genesis and Exodus of NOW, Second Edition* (self-pub., CreateSpace, 2014), 3.

15. Scribner, "Progress versus Tradition in Mobile," 177.

16. Alsobrook, "Alabama's Port City," 168.

17. Alsobrook, "Alabama's Port City," 179.

18. James C. Cobb, "World War II and the Mind of the Modern South," in *Remaking Dixie: The Impact of World War II on the Modern South*, ed. Neil R. McMillen (Jackson: University Press of Mississippi, 1997), 14.

19. Allen Cronenberg, "Mobile and World War II, 1940–1945," in Thomason, *Mobile*, 225.

20. Cronenberg, "Mobile and World War II," 223.

21. Quoted in Cronenberg, "Mobile and World War II," 225.

22. Kevern Verney, "'Every Man Should Try': John L. LeFlore and the National Association for the Advancement of Colored People in Alabama, 1919–1956," *Alabama Review* 66, no. 3 (2013): 186–210, https://doi.org/10.1353/ala.2013.0018.

23. Frye Gaillard, *Cradle of Freedom: Alabama and the Movement That Changed America* (Tuscaloosa: University of Alabama Press, 2004), 19.

24. Kristen Hannum, "How Father Albert Foley Took on the KKK," *U.S. Catholic* 78, no. 11 (2013): 47–48.

25. Hannum, "How Father Albert."

26. Brendan Kirby, "Mobile Press-Register 200th Anniversary: The Klan, Accommodation and the Battle for Mobile's Soul (1950–1959)," *Press-Register*, June 26, 2013, https://www.al.com/live/2013/06/mobile_press-register_200th_an_27.html.

27. Jim McDermott, "A Professor, a President and the Klan," *America Magazine*, April 16, 2007, https://www.americamagazine.org/politics-society/2007/04/16/professor-president-and-klan.

28. Gentry Holbert, "A Historical Moment: Spring Hill College," *Conversations on Jesuit Higher Education*, 2016, https://conversationsmagazine.org/a-historical-moment-spring-hill-college-b139210b5f32.

29. Roy Hoffman, *Back Home: Journeys through Mobile* (Tuscaloosa: University of Alabama Press, 2001), 252.

30. Hoffman, *Back Home*, 252.

31. Fredrick Douglas Richardson, *The Genesis and Exodus of NOW* (self-pub., CreateSpace, 2014), 36.

32. Richardson, *The Genesis and Exodus of NOW*, 34.

33. Interview with Fred Richardson and Noble Beasley, February 13, 2014 (Mobile: Fox10 News, 2021).

34. Dan Baum, "Legalize It All: How to Win the War on Drugs," *Harper's Magazine*, April 2016, https://harpers.org/archive/2016/04/legalize-it-all/.

35. Sonnie Wellington Hereford and Jack D. Ellis, *Beside the Troubled Waters: A Black Doctor Remembers Life, Medicine, and Civil Rights in an Alabama Town* (Tuscaloosa: University of Alabama Press, 2011), 144–49.

36. William Perry Fidler, *Augusta Evans Wilson, 1835–1909: A Biography* (Tuscaloosa: University of Alabama Press, 1951), 87.

37. Mobile Infirmary, "History," Infirmary Health (Mobile: Mobile Infirmary, 2021), https://www.infirmaryhealth.org/about/history.
38. Mary Ellen Maatman, "Speaking Truth to Memory: Lawyers and Resistance to the End of White Supremacy," *Howard Law Journal* 50, no. 1 (2006): 20.
39. Anthony Lewis, *Make No Law: The Sullivan Case and the First Amendment* (New York: Random House, 1991).
40. Four Alabama civil rights ministers (Reverends Ralph Abernathy, Joseph Lowery, Solomon Seay, and Fred Shuttlesworth) became casualties in this legal battle with the *Times*. Their names had been included as signatories of the advertisement without their knowledge or permission. They were added as the Alabama defendants in the libel suits and their automobiles and property were confiscated. See Jeffrey Toobin. "Keeping Speech Robust and Free," *New York Review of Books*, July 20, 2023: 27-29, https://www.nybooks.com/articles/2023/07/20/keeping-speech-robust-and-free-new-york-times-v-sullivan.
41. Quoted in Lewis, *Make No Law*, 25.
42. Jeremy W. Peters, "*Sarah Palin v. New York Times* Spotlights Push to Loosen Libel Law," *New York Times*, January 23, 2022, https://www.nytimes.com/2022/01/23/business/media/sarah-palin-libel-suit-nyt.html.
43. New York Times, "Robert Shelton, 73, Leader of Big Klan Faction," *New York Times*, March 20, 2003, https://www.nytimes.com/2003/03/20/us/robert-shelton-73-leader-of-big-klan-faction.html.
44. Morris Dees and Steve Fiffer, *Hate on Trial: The Case against America's Most Dangerous Neo-Nazi* (New York: Villard Books, 1993).
45. Southern Poverty Law Center, "Composite Complaint: Donald v. United Klan of America," 1985, https://www.splcenter.org/sites/default/files/d6_legacy_files/downloads/case/beulahvunklan_compcomplaint.pdf.
46. Morris Dees and Steve Fiffer, *A Lawyer's Journey: The Morris Dees Story* (Chicago: American Bar Association, 2001), 311–31.
47. "Robert Shelton, 73, Leader of Big Klan Faction," *New York Times*, March 20, 2003, https://www.nytimes.com/2003/03/20/us/robert-shelton-73-leader-of-big-klan-faction.html.
48. "Robert Shelton," *New York Times*, March 20, 2003.
49. Jefferson Cowie, *Freedom's Dominion* (New York: Basic Books, 2022), 290–93.
50. Peggy Wallace Kennedy and H. Mark Kennedy, *The Broken Road: George Wallace and a Daughter's Journey to Reconciliation* (New York: Bloomsbury Publishing, 2019), 127.
51. Kennedy and Kennedy, *Broken Road*, 162.
52. Scotty E. Kirkland, "Mobile and the Boswell Amendment," *Alabama Review* 65, no. 3 (July 2012): 214.
53. Kirkland, "Mobile and the Boswell Amendment," 214.
54. NAACP LDF, "Landmark: *Smith v. Allwright*" (New York: NAACP LDF, 2021), https://www.naacpldf.org/case-issue/landmark-smith-v-allwright.
55. Scotty E. Kirkland, "Mobile and the Boswell Amendment," *Alabama Review* 65, no. 3 (July 2012): 205–49; "Voting in the South," *Life*, May 15, 1944, 32–40.
56. Quoted in Kirkland, "Mobile and the Boswell Amendment," 227.
57. Quoted in Kirkland, "Mobile and the Boswell Amendment," 231.

58. Keith Nicholls, "Politics and Civil Rights in Post-World War II Mobile," in Thomason, *Mobile*, 253.

59. Scotty E. Kirkland, "Boswell Amendment," Encyclopedia of Alabama, 2018, http://www.encyclopediaofalabama.org/article/h-3085.

60. Kirkland, "Mobile and the Boswell Amendment."

61. While Alabama's electoral process is no longer subjected to federal oversight, a Supreme Court decision in 2023 appears to have unexpectedly prevented gerrymandering by Alabama's Republican-controlled legislature, which had limited Black voters' control to only one of Alabama's seven Congressional seats even though they represent about 25 percent of its population. The battle to preserve remnants of the Voting Rights Act of 1965 continues. See Nina Totenberg, "Supreme Court Unexpectedly Upholds Provision Prohibiting Racial Gerrymandering," National Public Radio, June 8, 2023. https://www.npr.org/2023/06/08/1181002182/supreme-court-voting-rights.

62. Richard A. Pride, *The Political Use of Racial Narratives: School Desegregation in Mobile, Alabama, 1954–97* (Urbana: University of Illinois Press, 2002), 26–28.

63. Richard A. Pride, *The Confession of Dorothy Danner* (Nashville, TN: Vanderbilt University Press, 1995), 251–57.

64. Brian Andrew Duke, "The Strange Career of Birdie Mae Davis: A History of a School Desegregation Lawsuit in Mobile, Alabama, 1963–1997," Department of History, Auburn University, 2009, https://etd.auburn.edu/bitstream/handle/10415/1654/Final Thesis.pdf.

65. Quoted in Erica Frankenberg, "The Impact and Limits of Implementing *Brown*: Reflections from Sixty-Five Years of School Segregation and Desegregation in Alabama's Largest School District," *Alabama Civil Rights and Civil Liberties Law Review* 11, no. 33 (2019): 6.

66. Feldman, *The Disfranchisement Myth: Poor Whites and Suffrage Restriction in Alabama*, 2004.

67. Heather McGhee, *The Sum of Us: What Racism Costs Everyone and How We Can Prosper Together* (New York: Random House, 2021).

68. Michael Meltsner, *The Making of a Civil Rights Lawyer* (Charlottesville: University of Virginia Press, 2006), 5–16.

69. Simpkins as quoted in David B. Smith, *Health Care Divided: Race and Healing a Nation* (Ann Arbor: University of Michigan Press, 1999), 90.

CHAPTER 6

1. Joy HP Harriman, *Health Care in Mobile: An Oral History of the 1940s* (self-pub., CreateSpace, 2011), 61–78.

2. The author is indebted to Bruce Williams, archivist for University History at Michigan, for the details related to Franklin's experiences in Ann Arbor.

3. "Michigan Third in Negro Enrollment," *Michigan Daily*, December 1, 1912, https://digital.bentley.umich.edu/midaily/mdp.39015071755669/226.

4. Quoted in Harriman, *Health Care in Mobile*, 67.

5. "Franklin Primary Health Center, Inc., History," Franklin Primary Health Center, 2021, https://franklinprimary.org/history.

6. "Health Center Program Impact and Growth," Health Resources and Services Administration, Health Center Program, December 2020, https://bphc.hrsa.gov/about/healthcenterprogram/index.html.
7. "Taped Interview with Dr. Sam Eichold," May 6, 1998, Smith Hospital Segregation Files.
8. Harriman, *Health Care in Mobile*.
9. Harriman, *Health Care in Mobile*, 100.
10. Sister Maria, "History of St. Martin de Porres Hospital, Mobile, Alabama," *Journal of the National Medical Association* 56, no. 4 (1964): 304.
11. Sister Maria, "History of St. Martin," 304.
12. Karen Kruse Thomas, *Deluxe Jim Crow: Civil Rights and American Health Policy, 1935–1954* (Athens: University of Georgia Press, 2011).

CHAPTER 7

1. "Dr. Elsie Jean Cowsert," Find a Grave, added June 5, 2009, https://www.findagrave.com/memorial/37974821/elsie-jean-cowsert.
2. Pensacola News Journal, "Williams-Cowsert Wedding in Mobile," *Pensacola New Journal*, March 29, 1916.
3. "Aunt Jane's Letter Club," *Times-Picayune: Young People's Paper*, April 7, 1935.
4. "Prize Movie Synopsis: 'When Destry Rides Again,'" *Times-Picayune: Young People's Paper*, October 12, 1940.
5. "Six Women Best Males as Medical School Opens," *Times-Picayune*, January 2, 1955.
6. David L. Good, *Orvie, the Dictator of Dearborn: The Rise and Reign of Orville L. Hubbard* (Detroit, MI: Wayne State University Press, 1989).
7. Good, *Orvie, the Dictator of Dearborn*, 31.
8. See Margaret A. Burnham, *By Hands Now Known: Jim Crow's Legal Executioners* (New York: W. W. Norton, 2022), 10-29.
9. "Dr. Charles Watts Taped Interview," August 28, 1996, Smith Hospital Segregation Files.
10. Coreil, interview with author, 2017, Smith Hospital Segregation Files.
11. Coreil, interview with author, 2017, Smith Hospital Segregation Files.
12. "Telephone Interview with Sister Mary John Code," September 5, 2017, Smith Hospital Segregation Files.
13. "Notes from Earl B. Wert Interview," 1998, Smith Hospital Segregation Files.
14. Harriman, *Health Care in Mobile*.
15. Vivian Cannon, "Providence State's First Hospital in International Comparisons," *Mobile Press-Register*, 1966.
16. E. Cowsert, "A Modern Health Program: Methods and Objectives," *Linacre Quarterly* 32, no. 2 (May 1, 1965), https://epublications.marquette.edu/lnq/vol32/iss2/13.
17. Cowsert, "A Modern Health Program," 157.
18. "Telephone Interview with Sister Mary John Code," September 5, 2017, Smith Hospital Segregation Files.
19. "Telephone Interview with Sister Mary John Code," September 5, 2017, Smith Hospital Segregation Files.

CHAPTER 8

1. Smith, *Health Care Divided*, 78–95.
2. David Barton Smith, "Forgotten Heroes: Remembering Dr. Alvin Blount, Who Helped Integrate America's Hospitals," *Health Affairs Blog*, September 1, 2017, https://www.healthaffairs.org/do/10.1377/hblog20170901.061774/full.
3. Kenneth L. Wilson et al., "The Forgotten MASH Surgeon: The Story of Alvin Vincent Blount Jr, MD," *Journal of the National Medical Association* 104, no. 3–4 (2012): 221–23.
4. Bernice Coreil, telephone interview, July 28, 2017, Smith Hospital Segregation Files.
5. "Taped Interview with Susan Chapman," September 9, 1995, Smith Hospital Segregation Files.
6. John L. LeFlore to James Quigley, "Letter to James Quigley," Non-Partisan Voter's League files, Archives of Southern Alabama University, March 24, 1965.
7. Joseph A. Califano Jr., *The Triumph and Tragedy of Lyndon Johnson: The White House Years* (New York: Simon and Schuster, 1991), 64–67.
8. Smith, *The Power to Heal*, 87–91.
9. NAACP Legal Defense Fund, "Report on Implementation of Title VI of the Civil Rights Act of 1964 in Regard to Hospital Discrimination: Recommendations for 1966," Medical Committee for Human Rights Collection (Philadelphia: University of Pennsylvania Library Archives, December 16, 1965).
10. "Notes from Follow-up Telephone Interview with Peter Libassi," August 10, 2015, Smith Hospital Segregation Files.
11. Peter Libassi to Cater, Katzenbach, and Califano, "Memo to Joseph Califano, Douglass Cater and Nicholas Katzenbach," May 6, 1966, Lyndon Baines Johnson Presidential Library and Museum, Austin, Texas (hereafter LBJ Library).
12. Douglass Cater, "Memo to the President, May 19, 1966," Box 14, Office Files of Douglass Cater, LBJ Library.
13. Farris Bryant to Lyndon B. Johnson, "Memorandum to the President, May," 1966, LBJ Library.
14. Lyndon Baines Johnson, "Remarks to Members of the National Council of Senior Citizens," *Public Papers of the Presidents of the United States: Lyndon B. Johnson (1966, Book 2)*, 578 [253] (Washington DC: Government Printing Office, 1966).
15. Lyndon Baines Johnson, "Remarks at a Meeting with Medical and Hospital Leaders to Prepare for the Launching of Medicare," *Public Papers of the Presidents of the United States: Lyndon B. Johnson (1966, Book 2)*, 605 [271] (Washington DC: Government Printing Office, 1966).
16. "Notes from Follow-up Telephone Interview with Peter Libassi," August 10, 2015, Smith Hospital Segregation Files.
17. The logic for exempting physicians receiving payment from Part B of Medicare from Title VI compliance was strained and is hard to explain. That a physician in private practice could receive Medicare payments under Part B, even if that practice included racially segregated waiting rooms, while a hospital clinic, paid for by Part A of Medicare could not, at least on the surface doesn't make much sense. The official explanation is that the 1964 Civil Rights bill, as a concession to Southern legislators, inserted the following exemption in Title VI: "Nothing in

this subchapter shall add or detract from any existing authority with respect to any program or activity under which federal financial assistance is extended by way of a contract of insurance or guaranty." The original intent of this exemption was to prevent Title VI being used to attack discriminatory housing by applying it to federal support of home mortgages and to protection of bank deposits. Subsequent fair housing legislation eliminated the purpose of this exemption. Yet, that exemption for Part B remained in place technically until the passage of Obama's Affordable Care Act. DHEW's general counsel at the time of Medicare's passage argued that Part B represented an indemnity insurance policy of which cash payments were made directly to the beneficiary and such payments were excluded from Title VI coverage. The practical purpose of the Part B exemption was that it would have been an administrative nightmare to enforce and would encourage physicians not to participate.

18. Young, interview with author, 1997, Smith Hospital Segregation Files.
19. Everett A. Johnson, "The Civil Rights Act of 1964—What It Means for Hospitals," *Hospitals* 38, (November 16, 1964): 53–54.
20. "Medical Society Protest," *Mobile Register*, December 14, 1966.
21. "Protest Letter," *Mobile Register*, December 17, 1966.
22. "Immoral Act Term Used by Governor," *Mobile Register*, December 20, 1966.
23. "Editorial," *Mobile Register*, December 18, 1966.
24. "Providence Expansion Announced," *Mobile Register*, December 21, 1966.
25. "City's Major Hospitals Await Medicare Approval," *Mobile Register*, June 28, 1966.
26. "No Hospital Rule," *Mobile Register*, January 6, 1967.
27. "No Hospital Rule," *Mobile Register*, January 6, 1967.
28. "Infirmary Issue Said Presented Inadequately," *Mobile Register*, February 8, 1967.
29. Paul Plotz, Interview with Dr. Paul Plotz, NIH, March 10, 2000, Personal Papers of Dr. Plotz.
30. *Mobile Register*, "Medicare Fight Won by Hospital," February 23, 1967.

CHAPTER 9

1. Angela D'Adamo et al., "Health Disparities in Past Influenza Pandemics: A Scoping Review of the Literature," *SSM - Population Health* 21, (March 2023).
2. Vanessa Northington Gamble, "There Wasn't a Lot of Comfort in Those Days," *Public Health Reports* 125, Suppl. 3 (2010), 114–22.
3. Anna M. Acosta et al., "Racial and Ethnic Disparities in Rates of COVID-19–Associated Hospitalization, Intensive Care Unit Admission, and In-Hospital Death in the United States from March 2020 to February 2021," *JAMA Network Open* 4, no. 10 (2021), e20134079.
4. Scotty E. Kirkland, *We the People* (Montgomery: Alabama Department of Archives and History, 2019): 89–90.
5. Matthew Desmond, *Poverty, by America* (New York: Crown, 2023), 188.
6. Desmond, *Poverty, by America*.
7. Jerry Mitchell, *Race Against Time* (New York: Simon and Schuster, 2019), 385–86.
8. Kyle Whitmire, "State of Denial: How 155 Angry White Men Chained Alabama to Its Confederate Past," AL.com, December 5, 2022, https://www.al.com/

news/2022/12/the-curse-of-1901-how-155-angry-white-men-chained-alabama-to-its-confederate-past.html.

9. Equal Justice Initiative, *Lynching in America: Confronting the Legacy of Racial Terror*, 3rd ed. (Montgomery, AL: Equal Justice Initiative, 2017), https//eji.org/rerports/lynching-in-america.

10. United States Department of Justice, "The Attorney General's Second Annual Report to Congress Pursuant to the Emmett Till Unsolved Civil Rights Crime Act of 2007," May 13, 2010, https://www.justice.gov/sites/default/files/crt/legacy/2015/06/18/tillreport_02.pdf.

11. United States Department of Justice, "The Attorney General's Ninth Annual Report to Congress Pursuant to the Emmett Till Unsolved Civil Rights Crime Act of 2007 and Third Annual Report to Congress Pursuant to the Emmett Till Unsolved Civil Rights Crimes Reauthorization Act of 2016," March 1, 2021, 18 https://www.justice.gov/crt/file/1405431/download.

12. Doug Jones, *Bending Toward Justice* (New York: Simon and Schuster, 2019).

13. Jerry Mitchell, *Race Against Time* (New York: Simon and Schuster, 2019).

14. Samantha Michaels, "A Jim Crow-Era Murder. A Family Secret. Decades Later, What Does Justice Look Like?," *Mother Jones* (San Francisco: Foundation for National Progress, December 2021), https:/www.motherjones.com/politics/2021/10/jim-crow-unsolved-murder-lynching-justice-margaret-burnham-stories-families.

15. Civil Rights and Restorative Justice Project, "Incidents Which Took Place in Mobile, AL," database report (January 2022).

16. See Davis Video: CRRJ Project, "Murder in Mobile." Northeastern University School of Law, posted August 8, 2019, https://www.youtube.com/watch?v=KwP-HdBrYjo.

17. Scotty Kirkland, telephone interview, August 25, 2020, Smith Hospital Segregation Files.

18. Medical Society of Mobile County, "Memorial Resolution for Dr. Elsie Jean Cowsert" (Birmingham, AL: University of Alabama Birmingham, February 21, 1967).

19. There are now 161 on this list. The DOJ discloses information on cases only after they are closed. Andrew Goodman and Michael Schwerner are among the eight whites in closed cases on the list. They were volunteers in a voter registration drive and victims of Klan members in Philadelphia, Mississippi, on June 21, 1964. Two Black physicians, Dr. George Washington Singleton Jr., of Shelby, North Carolina, and Dr. Thomas Brewer, founder of the local chapter of the NAACP in Columbus, Georgia, are closed cases on this list. Seven women are also included among the closed cases. As of April 2022, 26 of these cases, including Dr. Cowsert's, remain open.

20. Department of Justice, "Cases Opened under the Till Act and Its Reauthorization" (Civil Rights Section, Criminal Division, 2022), https://www.justice.gov/crt/page/file/1470121/download.

21. George Washington Law Review, "Title VI of the Civil Rights Act of 1964: Implementation and Impact," *George Washington Law Review* 36 (1968), 989.

22. "Taped Interview with Frank Weil," May 26, 1995, Smith Hospital Segregation Files.

23. Bobby Childers and Vanessa Burrows, "Taped Interview with Bobby Childers," produced by Barbara Berney (BLB Productions, Jan. 4, 2014).

24. Elizabeth H. Cobbs and Petric J. Smith, *Long Time Coming: An Insider's Story of the Birmingham Church Bombing That Rocked the World* (Birmingham, AL: Crane Hill, 1994), 64–65.

25. David Barton Smith, "The Racial Segregation of Hospital Care Revisited: Medicare Discharge Patterns and Their Implications," *American Journal of Public Health* 88, no. 3 (1998): 461–63. https://doi.org/10.2105/AJPH.88.3.461.

26. Howard Zinn, *You Can't Be Neutral on a Moving Train* (Boston: Beacon Press, 1995).

27. Desmond Tutu, "Remembering," 2022, https://www.azquotes.com/quote/380816.

28. Ronald M. Davis, "Achieving Racial Harmony for the Benefit of Patients and Communities: Contrition, Reconciliation, and Collaboration," *JAMA* 300, no. 3 (July 16, 2008), 323–25, https://doi.org/10.1001/jama.300.3.323.

29. David Barton Smith, "Forgotten Heroes: Remembering Dr. Alvin Blount, Who Helped Integrate America's Hospitals." *Health Affairs Blog*, September 1, 2017, https//www.healthaffairs.org/do/101877/hblog20170901.061774/full.

30. Gabrielle Redford, "AAMC Renames Prestigious Abraham Flexner Award in Light of Racist and Sexist Writings," Association of American Medical Colleges, Nov. 17, 2020, https://www.aamc.org/news-insights/aamc-renames-prestigious-abraham-flexner-award-light-racist-and-sexist-writings.

31. Kevin A. Schulman, Jesse A. Berlin, William Harless, et al., "The Effect of Race and Sex on Physicians' Recommendations for Cardiac Catheterization," *New England Journal of Medicine* 340 (1999), 618–26.

32. Romana Hasnain-Wynia et al., "Disparities in Health Care Are Driven by Where Minority Patients Seek Care: Examination of the Hospital Quality Alliance Measures," *Archives of Internal Medicine* 167, no. 12 (June 25, 2007), 1233–39, https://doi.org/10.1001/archinte.167.12.1233.

33. Richard D. deShazo, Craig J. Hoesley, and Selwyn M. Vickers, "Ending Racial Bias in American Medicine: A Call for Help from the AMA, NMA, AAMC, and the Rest of Us," *American Journal of Medicine* 134, no. 5 (May 2021), 565–68, https://doi.org/10.1016/j.amjmed.2020.11.011.

34. David A. Acosta and David J. Skorton, "Making 'Good Trouble': Time for Organized Medicine to Call for Racial Justice in Medical Education and Health Care," *American Journal of Medicine* 134, no. 10 (2021): 1203–9; Aletha Maybank et al., "Embedding Racial Justice and Advancing Health Equity at the American Medical Association," *American Journal of Medicine* 135, no. 7 (July 2022), 803–5, https://doi.org/10.1016/j.amjmed.2022.01.058.

35. Kenneth M. Ludmerer, *Time to Heal: American Medical Education from the Turn of the Century to Managed Care* (New York: Oxford University Press, 1999): 283.

36. AAMC, "Revenue by Source, FY 1977 through FY 2022," Association of American Medical Colleges, copyright 2023, https://www.aamc.org/data-reports/data/iv-revenue-source-fy-1977-through-fy-2022.

37. Arnold S. Relman, "The New Medical-Industrial Complex," *New England Journal of Medicine* 303, no. 11 (1980): 963–70.

38. Dayna Bowen Matthew, *Just Medicine: A Cure for Racial Inequality in American Health Care* (New York: New York University Press, 2015), 27.

39. Matthew, *Just Medicine*, 210–11.

40. Nisha Agarwal, "Complaint of Health REACH Pursuant to Title VI of the Civil Rights Act of 1964, The Hill Burton Act, The New York State Patients' Bill of Rights and the New York City Human Rights Law" (New York Lawyers for the Public Interest Inc. (2008), https://www.nylpi.org/images/FE/chain234siteType8/site203/client/COMPLAINT-FINAL-FULL.pdf.

41. Jack Geiger as quoted in Bill Lubinger, "Dialogue: A Public Health Pioneer," *Think: The Online Magazine of Case Western Reserve* (2021), https://case.edu/think/spring2016/public-health-pioneer.html.

42. Sonya V. Troller-Renfree et al., "The Impact of a Poverty Reduction Intervention on Infant Brain Activity," *PNAS* 119, no. 5 (2022), e2115649119 (1–8).

43. Andrew C. Barr, Jonathan Eggleston, and Alexander A. Smith, "Investing in Infants: The Lasting Effects of Cash Transfers to New Families," *Quarterly Journal of Economics*, 137, no. 44 (2022): 2539–83.

44. McGhee, *The Sum of Us.*

45. J. P. Mackenbach, "Politics Is Nothing but Medicine at a Larger Scale: Reflections on Public Health's Biggest Idea," *Journal of Epidemiology and Community Health* 63, no. 3 (2009), 181–84.

ACKNOWLEDGMENTS

1. See Smith, *The Power to Heal*, 200.

2. I had assumed that being involved in such lawsuits would be an isolating experience and found just the opposite. Many minority interest groups, some of whom I was unaware even existed, joined in support. Both defendants apparently welcomed the suits because it gave them leverage to work on the problems. The law firms representing the defendants welcomed it as a potential revenue-producing product line, putting on workshops to promote it. All the pieces of the system are well connected, and I enjoyed the opportunity to work with all of them.

3. Smith, *Health Care Divided.*

4. See Burnett, *Power to Heal: Medicare and the Civil Rights Revolution* (Bullfrog Films, 2018), http://bullfrogfilms.com/catalog/pth.html; Smith, *The Power to Heal.*

5. Harriman, *Health Care in Mobile.*

6. See, for example, Frye Gaillard, *Cradle of Freedom: Alabama and the Movement That Changed America* (Tuscaloosa: University of Alabama Press, 2004).

7. deShazo, *The Racial Divide in American Medicine.*

8. David Barton Smith, "The Pandemic Challenge: End Separate and Unequal Healthcare," *American Journal of Medical Sciences* 360, no. 2 (August 2020): 109–11.

9. Burnham, *By Hands Now Known: Jim Crow's Legal Executioners.*

BIBLIOGRAPHY

ARCHIVES

David Barton Smith Hospital Segregation Files, Charles L. Blockson Afro-American
Collection, Temple University Libraries, Philadelphia, Pennsylvania
Doy Leale McCall Rare Book and Manuscript Library, University of South Alabama,
Mobile, Alabama
Kislak Center for Special Collections, Rare Books and Manuscripts, University of
Pennsylvania, Philadelphia, Pennsylvania
Library of Social and Economic Aspects of Medicine of Michael M. Davis, The Drs.
Barry and Bobbi Coller Rare Book Room, New York Academy of Medicine
Library, New York, New York
Lyndon Baines Johnson Presidential Library and Museum, Austin, Texas

REFERENCES

Acosta, Anna M., Shikha Garg, Huong Pham, et al. "Racial and Ethnic Disparities in
Rates of COVID-19–Associated Hospitalization, Intensive Care Unit Admission,
and In-Hospital Death in the United States from March 2020 to February 2021."
JAMA Network Open 4, no. 10 (2021): 1–15.
Acosta, David A., and David J. Skorton. "Making 'Good Trouble': Time for Organized
Medicine to Call for Racial Justice in Medical Education and Health Care." *American Journal of Medicine* 134, no. 10 (2021): 1203–09.
Agarwal, Nisha. "Complaint of Health Reach Pursuant to Title VI of the Civil Rights
Act of 1964, the Hill Burton Act, the New York State Patients' Bill of Rights, and
the New York City Human Rights Law." New York Lawyers for the Public Interest,
June 9, 2008. https://www.nylpi.org/images/FE/chain234siteType8/site203/client/
COMPLAINT-FINAL-FULL.pdf.
Alexander, Michelle. *The New Jim Crow: Mass Incarceration in the Age of Colorblindness.* New York: The New Press, 2010.
Alsobrook, David Ernest. "Alabama's Port City: Mobile During the Progressive Era,
1896–1917." PhD diss., Auburn University, 1983.
Altmeyer, Arthur J. *The Formative Years of Social Security.* Madison: University of
Wisconsin Press, 1966.
Ascoli, Peter M. *Julius Rosenwald: The Man Who Built Sears, Roebuck and Advanced
the Cause of Black Education in the American South.* Bloomington: Indiana
University Press, 2006.

Bahr, Sarah. "Roosevelt Statue to Head to Presidential Library in North Dakota." *New York Times*, November 19, 2021. https://www.nytimes.com/2021/11/19/arts/design/roosevelt-statue-north-dakota.html.

Barr, Andrew C., Jonathan Eggleston, and Alexander A. Smith. 2022. "Investing in Infants: The Lasting Effects of Cash Transfers to New Families." *Quarterly Journal of Economics* 137, no. 4 (August 2022): 2539–83.

Barry, John M. *The Great Influenza: The Story of the Deadliest Pandemic in History.* New York: Random House, 2018.

Baum, Dan. "Legalize It All: How to Win the War on Drugs." *Harper's Magazine*, April 1, 2016. https://harpers.org/archive/2016/04/legalize-it-all.

Beck, Andrew H. "The Flexner Report and the Standardization of American Medical Education." *JAMA* 291, no. 17 (May 2004): 2139–40.

Beckert, Sven, and Seth Rockman. *Slavery's Capitalism: A New History of American Economic Development.* Philadelphia: University of Pennsylvania Press, 2016.

Beito, David T. "The 'Lodge Practice Evil' Reconsidered: Medical Care through Fraternal Societies, 1900–1930." *Journal of Urban History* 23, no. 5 (July 1997): 569–600.

Berliner, Howard S. "A Larger Perspective on the Flexner Report." *International Journal of Health Services: Planning, Administration, Evaluation* 5, no. 4 (1975): 573–90. https://doi.org/10.2190/F31Q-592N-056K-VETL.

Best, Matthew J., Edward G. McFarland, Savyasachi C. Thakkar, and Uma Srikumaran. "Racial Disparities in the Use of Surgical Procedures in the US." *JAMA Surgery* 156, no. 3 (March 2021): 274–81.

Blackmon, Douglas A. *Slavery by Another Name: The Re-Enslavement of Black Americans from the Civil War to World War II.* New York: Anchor Books, 2008.

Brace, C. Loring. "The 'Ethnology' of Josiah Clark Nott." *Bulletin of the New York Academy of Medicine* 50, no. 4 (April 1974): 509–28.

Brueske, Paul. *The Last Siege: The Mobile Campaign, Alabama 1865.* Philadelphia, PA: Casemate, 2018.

Burnett, Charles, and David Lowenthal, producers. *Power to Heal: Medicare and the Civil Rights Revolution.* BLB Film Productions, 2015.

Burnham, Margaret A. *By Hands Now Known: Jim Crow's Legal Executioners.* New York: W. W. Norton, 2022.

Califano, Joseph A., Jr. *The Triumph and Tragedy of Lyndon Johnson: The White House Years.* New York: Simon and Schuster, 1991.

Cannon, Vivian. "Providence Stater's First Hospital in International Comparisons." *Mobile Press-Register*, 1966.

Carson, Clayborne, David Garrow, Bill Kovach, and Carol Polsgrove. *Reporting Civil Rights: American Journalism 1941–1963.* 2 vols. New York: Library of America, 2003.

Case, Anne, and Angus Deaton. *Deaths of Despair and the Future of Capitalism.* Princeton, NJ: Princeton University Press, 2020.

Childers, Bobby, and Vanessa Burrows. "Taped Interview with Bobby Childers." Produced by Barbara Berney. BLB Productions, Jan. 4, 2014.

Civil Rights and Restorative Justice Project. "Murder in Mobile." Northeastern University School of Law. 2022. Murder in Mobile. YouTube video, 23:36. https://www.youtube.com/watch?v=KwP-HdBrYjo.

Clements, Kendrick A. *The Presidency of Woodrow Wilson.* Lawrence: University Press of Kansas, 1992.

Cobb, James C. "World War II and the Mind of the Modern South." In *Remaking Dixie: The Impact of World War II on the American South,* edited by Neil R. McMillen, 14–22. Jackson: University Press of Mississippi, 1997.

Cobb, W. Montague. "Surgery and the Negro Physician: Some Parallels in Background." *Journal of the National Medical Association* 43, no.3 (May 1951): 145–52.

Cobbs, Elizabeth H., and Petric J. Smith. *Long Time Coming: An Insider's Story of the Birmingham Church Bombing That Rocked the World.* Birmingham, AL: Crane Hill, 1994.

Cohen, Alan B., David C. Colby, Keith A. Wailoo, and Julian E. Zelizer, eds. *Medicare and Medicaid at 50: America's Entitlement Programs in the Age of Affordable Care.* New York: Oxford University Press, 2015.

"The Committee on the Costs of Medical Care." *JAMA* 99, no. 23 (1932): 1950–52.

Cowie, Jefferson. *Freedom's Dominion.* New York: Basic Books, 2022.

Cowsert, Eleanor Jean. "A Modern Health Program: Methods and Objectives." *Linacre Quarterly* 32, no. 2 (May 1965): 157–59.

Cronenberg, Allen. "Mobile and World War II, 1940–1945." In Thomason, *Mobile,* 209–46.

D'Adamo, Angela, Alina Schnake-Mahl, Pricila H. Mullachery, Mariana Lazo, Ana V. Diez Roux, and Usama Bilal. "Health Disparities in Past Influenza Pandemics: A Scoping Review of the Literature." *SSM - Population Health,* no. 21 (March 2023).

Davis, Loyal. *Fellowship of Surgeons: A History of the American College of Surgeons.* Chicago: American College of Surgeons, 1960.

Davis, Ronald M. "Achieving Racial Harmony for the Benefit of Patients and Communities: Contrition, Reconciliation, and Collaboration." *JAMA* 300, no. 3 (2008): 323–25. https://doi.org/10.1001/jama.300.3.323.

Dees, Morris, and Steve Fiffer. *Hate on Trial: The Case against America's Most Dangerous Neo-Nazi.* New York: Villard Books, 1993.

———. *A Lawyer's Journey: The Morris Dees Story.* Chicago: American Bar Association, 2001.

Delgado, James P., Deborah E. Marx, Kyle Lent, Joseph Grinnan, and Alexander DeCaro. Clotilda: *The History and Archaeology of the Last Slave Ship.* Tuscaloosa: University of Alabama Press, 2023.

Department of Justice. "Cases Opened under the Till Act and Its Reauthorization." Civil Rights Section, Criminal Division, 2022. https://www.justice.gov/crt/file/1470121/download.

deShazo, Richard D., ed. *The Racial Divide in American Medicine: Black Physicians and the Struggle for Justice in Health Care.* Jackson: University Press of Mississippi, 2018.

deShazo, Richard D., Keydron K. Guinn, Wayne J. Riley, and William F. Winter. "A Crooked Path Made Straight: The Rise and Fall of the Southern Governors' Plan for Black Physicians (1945–1970)." In *The Racial Divide in American Medicine: Black Physicians and the Struggle for Justice in Health Care,* edited by Richard deShazo, 71–82. Jackson: University Press of Mississippi, 2018.

deShazo, Richard D., Craig J. Hosley, and Selwyn M. Vickers. "Ending Racial Bias in American Medicine: A Call for Help from the AMA, NMA, AAMC and the Rest of Us." *American Journal of Medicine* 134, no. 5 (May 2021): 565–68. https://doi.org/10.1016/j.amjmed.2020.11.011.

Desmond, Matthew. "Capitalism." In *The 1619 Project,* edited by Nikole Hannah-Jones, 165–185. New York: One World, 2021.

————. *Poverty, by America*. New York: Crown, 2023.

Diner, Hasia R. *Julius Rosenwald: Repairing the World*. New Haven, CT: Yale University Press, 2017.

Donabedian, Avedis. *Exploring Quality Assessment and Monitoring: The Definition of Quality and Approaches to Its Assessment. Vol. 1 Explorations in Quality Assessment and Monitoring*. Ann Arbor, MI: Health Administration Press, 1980.

"Donald v. United Klans of America: Case Number 84-0725." Southern Poverty Law Center, accessed July 13, 2023. https://www.splcenter.org/seeking-justice/case-docket/donald-v-united-klans-america.

Doss, Harriet E. Amos. "Cotton City, 1813–1860." In Thomason, *Mobile*.

Du Bois, W. E. B. *Black Reconstruction in America*. New York: Harcourt Brace, 1935.

Duffy, Thomas P. "The Flexner Report—100 Years Later." *Yale Journal of Biology and Medicine* 84, no. 3 (September 2011): 269–76.

Duke, Brian Andrew. "The Strange Career of Birdie Mae Davis: A History of a School Desegregation Lawsuit in Mobile, Alabama, 1963–1997." Master's thesis, Auburn University, 2009. https://etd.auburn.edu/bitstream/handle/10415/1654/Final Thesis.pdf.

Equal Justice Initiative. *Lynching in America: Confronting the Legacy of Racial Terror*, 3rd ed. Montgomery, AL: Equal Justice Initiative, 2017. https://eji.org/reports/lynching-in-america.

————. *Reconstruction in America: Racial Violence after the Civil War: 1865–1876*. Montgomery, AL: Equal Justice Initiative, 2020. https://eji.org/report/reconstruction-in-america.

Falk, Isidore Sydney, Margaret Klem, and Nathan Sinai. "The Incidence of Illness and the Receipt and Costs of Medical Care among Representative Families." Publications of the Committee on the Cost of Medical Care, no. 26. Chicago: University of Chicago Press, 1932.

Feldman, Glenn. *The Disfranchisement Myth: Poor Whites and Suffrage Restriction in Alabama*. Athens: University of Georgia Press, 2004.

Fidler, William Perry. *Augusta Evans Wilson, 1835–1909: A Biography*. Tuscaloosa: University of Alabama Press, 1951. ebook.

Field, Robert I. *The Mother of Invention: How the Government Created "Free Market" Health Care*. New York: Oxford University Press, 2014.

Fioretos, Orfeo, Tulia G. Falleti, and Adam Sheingate. *The Oxford Handbook of Historical Institutionalism*. Oxford: Oxford University Press, 2016.

Fitzgerald, Michael W. *Urban Emancipation: Popular Politics in Reconstruction Mobile, 1860–1890*. Baton Rouge: Louisiana State University Press, 2002.

Fitzpatrick, Frank. "My Great-Grandfather Was a Mortician during the 1918–19 Flu Pandemic, and Bodies Filled His House." *Philadelphia Inquirer*, April 28, 2020, https://www.inquirer.com/news/coronavirus-spanish-flu-1918-philadelphia-camac-mortician-funeral-home-20200428.html.

Flexner, Abraham. *Medical Education in the United States and Canada: A Report to the Carnegie Foundation for the Advancement of Teaching*. New York: Carnegie Foundation for the Advancement of Teaching, 1910. http://archive.carnegiefoundation.org/publications/pdfs/elibrary/Carnegie_Flexner_Report.pdf.

Frankenberg, Erica. "The Impact and Limits of Implementing *Brown*: Reflections from Sixty-Five Years of School Segregation and Desegregation in Alabama's Largest District." *Alabama Civil Rights and Civil Liberties Law Review* 11, no. 1 (2019): 33–112.

Gaillard, Frye. *Cradle of Freedom: Alabama and the Movement that Changed America.* Tuscaloosa: University of Alabama Press, 2004.

Gamble, Vanessa Northington. *Making a Place for Ourselves.* New York: Oxford University Press, 1995.

———. "There Wasn't a Lot of Comfort in Those Days." *Public Health Reports* 125, Suppl. 3 (2010): 114–22.

Gayle, Caleb. "100 Years after the Tulsa Massacre, What Does Justice Look Like?" *New York Times Magazine,* May 25, 2021. https://www.nytimes.com/2021/05/25/magazine/tulsa-race-massacre-1921-greenwood.html.

George Washington Law Review. "Title VI of the Civil Rights Act of 1964: Implementation and Impact." *George Washington Law Review* 36 (1968): 824–1022.

Good, David L. *Orvie, the Dictator of Dearborn: The Rise and Reign of Orville L. Hubbard.* Detroit, MI: Wayne State University Press, 1989.

Gordon, Colin. *Dead on Arrival: The Politics of Health Care in Twentieth-Century America.* Princeton, NJ: Princeton University Press, 2004.

Gorman, Amanda. *The Hill We Climb: An Inaugural Poem for the Country.* New York: Viking, 2021.

Grantham-Philips, Wyatte. "On the Navajo Nation, COVID-19 Death Toll Is Higher than Any US State: Here's How You Can Support Community Relief." *USA TODAY,* October 24, 2020. https://www.usatoday.com/story/news/nation/2020/10/24/covid-native-americans-how-to-help-navajo-nation/3652816001.

Hall, Peter A. "Historical Institutionalism in Rationalist and Sociological Perspective." In *Explaining Institutional Change,* edited by James Mahoney and Kathleen Thelen. Cambridge: Cambridge University Press, 2010.

Hamowy, Ronald. "The Early Development of Medical Licensing Laws in the United States, 1875–1900." *Journal of Libertarian Studies* 3, no. 1 (1979): 73–149.

Hannum, Kristen. "How Father Albert Foley took on the KKK." *U.S. Catholic,* November 19, 2013. https://uscatholic.org/articles/201311/father-albert-foley-how-one-priest-took-on-the-kkk.

Harriman, Joy HP. *Health Care in Mobile: An Oral History of the 1940s.* Self-published, CreateSpace, 2011.

Hasnain-Wynia, Romana, David W. Baker, David Nerenz, Joe Feinglass, Anne C. Beal, Mary Beth Landrum, Raj Behal, and Joel S. Weissman. "Disparities in Health Care Are Driven by Where Minority Patients Seek Care: Examination of the Hospital Quality Alliance Measures." *Archives of Internal Medicine* 167, no. 12 (2007): 1233–39. https://doi.org/10.1001/archinte.167.12.1233.

Heen, Mary L. "Ending Jim Crow Life Insurance Rates." *Northwestern Journal of Law and Social Policy* 4, no. 2 (Fall 2009): 360–99.

Hereford, Sonnie Wellington, and Jack D. Ellis. *Beside the Troubled Waters: A Black Doctor Remembers Life, Medicine, and Civil Rights in an Alabama Town.* Tuscaloosa: University of Alabama Press, 2011.

Higginbotham, Jay. "Discovery, Exploration, and Colonization of Mobile to 1711." In Thomason, *Mobile.*

Hill, Karlos K. *Tulsa, 1921: Reporting a Massacre.* Norman: University of Oklahoma Press, 2019.

Hoffman, Beatrix. *Health Care for Some: Rights and Rationing in the United States since 1930.* Chicago: University of Chicago Press, 2012.

Hoffman, Frederick L. "Race Traits and Tendencies of the American Negro." *American Economic Association* 11, no. 1/3 (1896): 1–329.

Hoffman, Roy. *Back Home: Journeys through Mobile.* Tuscaloosa: University of Alabama Press, 2001.

Hollmuller, Anne. "The Dedication of the Lincoln Memorial." *Boundary Stones Blog*, April 18, 2018. https://boundarystones.weta.org/2018/04/18/dedication-lincoln-memorial.

Hotez, Peter J. *Preventing the Next Pandemic: Vaccine Diplomacy in a Time of Antiscience.* Baltimore, MD: Johns Hopkins University Press, 2021.

Hurston, Zora Neale. *Barracoon: The Story of the Last "Black Cargo."* New York: Amistad, 2018.

Institute on Taxation and Economic Policy. "Alabama State and Local Taxes." *Who Pays?: A Distributional Analysis of the Tax Systems in All 50 States*, 6th ed. Washington, DC: Institute on Taxation and Economic Policy, 2018. https://itep.sfo2.digitaloceanspaces.com/itep-whopays-Alabama.pdf.

Jager, Steven J. "Dyer Anti-Lynching Bill (1922)." Black Past, August 19, 2012. https://www.blackpast.org/african-american-history/dyer-anti-lynching-bill-1922.

Johnson, Everett A. "The Civil Rights Act of 1964—What It Means for Hospitals." *Hospitals*, no. 38 (November 16, 1964): 51–4.

Johnson, Lyndon Baines. "Remarks at a Meeting with Medical and Hospital Leaders to Prepare for the Launching of Medicare," *Public Papers of the Presidents of the United States: Lyndon B. Johnson (1966, Book 2)*, 605 [271]. Washington DC: Government Printing Office, 1966. https://www.cdc.gov/nchs/data/hus/2019/005–508.pdf.

———. "Remarks to Members of the National Council of Senior Citizens." *Public Papers of the Presidents of the United States: Lyndon B. Johnson (1966, Book 2)*, 578 [253]. Washington DC: Government Printing Office, 1966. https://www.cdc.gov/nchs/data/hus/2019/005–508.pdf.

Jones, Doug. *Bending Toward Justice: The Birmingham Church Bombing that Changed the Course of Civil Rights.* New York: Simon and Schuster, 2019.

Jones, James H. *Bad Blood: The Tuskegee Syphilis Experiment.* New York: Free Press, 1981.

Joynt, Karen E., E. John Orav, and Ashish K. Jha. "Thirty-Day Readmission Rates for Medicare Beneficiaries by Race and Site of Care." *JAMA* 305, no. 7 (February 2011): 475–681.

Kennedy, Peggy Wallace, and H. Mark Kennedy. *The Broken Road: George Wallace and a Daughter's Journey to Reconciliation.* New York: Bloomsbury Publishing, 2019.

Kirby, Brendan. "*Mobile Press-Register* 200th Anniversary: The Klan, Accommodation and the Battle for Mobile's Soul (1950–1959)." *Mobile Press-Register*, June 26, 2013. https://www.al.com/live/2013/06/mobile_press-register_200th_an_27.html.

Kirkland, Scotty E. "Boswell Amendment." Encyclopedia of Alabama. Last modified March 30, 2023. http://www.encyclopediaofalabama.org/article/h-3085.

———. "Mobile and the Boswell Amendment." *Alabama Review* 65, no. 3 (January 2012): 205–48.

———. *We the People.* Montgomery: Alabama Department of Archives and History, 2019.

Knox, John B. "Opening Remarks 1901 Proceedings of the Constitutional Convention, Day 2 of 54, Page 8." 1901. http://www.legislature.state.al.us/aliswww/history/constitutions/1901/proceedings/1901_proceedings_vol1/day2.html.

Koch, Alexander, Chris Brierley, Mark M. Maslin, and Simon L. Lewis. "Earth System Impacts of the European Arrival and the Great Dying in the Americas after 1492." *Quaternary Science Reviews* 207, no. 1 (March 2019): 13–36. https://doi.org/10.1016/j.quascirev.2018.12.004.

Krieger, Nancy, David H. Rehkopf, Jarvis T. Chen, Pamela D. Waterman, Enrico Marcelli, and Malinda Kennedy. "The Fall and Rise of US Inequities in Premature Mortality: 1960–2002." *PLOS Medicine* 5, no. 2 (2008): 227–40.

Kühl, Stefan. *The Nazi Connection: Eugenics, American Racism, and German National Socialism*. New York: Oxford University Press, 2002.

Laham, Nicholas. *Why the United States Lacks a National Health Insurance Program*. Westport, CT: Greenwood Press, 1993.

Lepore, Jill. "The Parent Trap." *New Yorker*, March 21, 2022, 16–21.

Lewis, Anthony. *Make No Law: The Sullivan Case and the First Amendment*. New York: Random House, 1991.

Lewis, David L. *W. E. B. Du Bois: A Biography*. New York: Holt Paperbacks, 2009.

Lincoln, Abraham. "Gettysburg Address." November 19, 1863. American Battlefield Trust, accessed June 26, 2023. https://www.battlefields.org/learn/primary-sources/abraham-lincolns-gettysburg-address.

Lubove, Roy. *The Struggle for Social Security, 1900–1935*. Cambridge, MA: Harvard University Press, 1968.

Ludmerer, Kenneth M. *Time to Heal: American Medical Education from the Turn of the Century to Managed Care*. New York: Oxford University Press, 1999.

Lyman, Brian. "Alabama Constitution: Committee Approves Plan to Remove Racist Language." *Montgomery Advertiser*, November 3, 2021, https://www.montgomeryadvertiser.com/story/news/2021/11/03/alabama-constitution-committee-approves-plan-remove-racist-language/6244819001.

Maatman, Mary Ellen. "Speaking Truth to Memory: Lawyers and Resistance to the End of White Supremacy." *Howard Law Journal* 50, no. 1 (2006): 8–45.

Mackenbach, J. P. "Politics Is Nothing but Medicine at a Larger Scale: Reflections on Public Health's Biggest Idea." *Journal of Epidemiology and Community Health* 63, no. 3 (March 2009): 181–84.

Matthew, Dayna Bowen. *Just Medicine: A Cure for Racial Inequality in American Health Care*. New York: New York University Press, 2015.

Maxwell, Angie, and Todd Shields. *The Long Southern Strategy: How Chasing White Voters in the South Changed American Politics*. New York: Oxford University Press, 2019.

Maybank, Aletha, Fernando De Maio, Diana Lemos, and Diana N. Derige. "Embedding Racial Justice and Advancing Health Equity at the American Medical Association." *American Journal of Medicine* 135, no. 7 (July 2022): 803–5. https://doi.org/10.1016/j.amjmed.2022.01.058.

McDermott, Jim. "A Professor, a President and the Klan." *America Magazine*, April 16, 2007, https://www.americamagazine.org/politics-society/2007/04/16/professor-president-and-klan.

McGhee, Heather. *The Sum of Us: What Racism Costs Everyone and How We Can Prosper Together*. New York: Random House, 2021.

McKiven, Henry M. "Secession, War, and Reconstruction, 1850–1874." In Thomason, *Mobile*, 95–126.

Meltsner, Michael. *The Making of a Civil Rights Lawyer*. Charlottesville: University of Virginia Press, 2006.

Michaels, Samantha. "A Jim Crow–Era Murder. A Family Secret. Decades Later, What Does Justice Look Like?" *Mother Jones*, November–December 2021. https://www.motherjones.com/politics/2021/10/jim-crow-unsolved-murder-lynching-justice-margaret-burnham-stories-families.

Mitchell, Jerry. *Race Against Time*. New York: Simon and Schuster, 2019.

Mitchell, Paul Wolff. "Black Philadelphians in the Samuel George Morton Cranial Collection." *Penn Arts and Sciences*, February 15, 2021, https://prss.sas.upenn.edu/penn-medicines-role/black-philadelphians-samuel-george-morton-cranial-collection.

"Mr. Trotter and Mr. Wilson." *The Crisis* 9, no. 3 (January 1915): 119–20.

Muhammad, Abdul-Aliy. "Laying Questions to Rest: Treatment of MOVE Remains Demands Probe." *Philadelphia Inquirer*, May 9, 2021. https://www.inquirer.com/opinion/commentary/move-remains-penn-museum-city-officials-temple-archives-20210505.html.

"Founding and Early Years," *NAACP: A Century in the Fight for Freedom*. Library of Congress, Exhibitions, 2021. https://www.loc.gov/exhibits/naacp/founding-and-early-years.html.

NAACP Legal Defense Fund. "Landmark: *Smith v. Allwright*." NAACP LDF, date filed November 10, 1943. https://www.naacpldf.org/case-issue/landmark-smith-v-allwright.

Nahrwold, David L., and Peter J. Kernahan. *A Century of Surgeons and Surgery*. Chicago: American College of Surgeons, 2012.

National Center for Health Statistics. *Health, United States, 2010*. Hyattsville, MD: Department of Health and Human Services, 2011. https://www.ncbi.nlm.nih.gov/books/NBK54381.

———. "Leading Causes of Death, 1900–1998." Centers for Disease Control and Prevention, accessed July 8, 2023. https://www.cdc.gov/nchs/data/dvs/lead1900_98.pdf.

———. "Table 5. Age-Adjusted Death Rates for Selected Causes of Death, by Sex, Race, and Hispanic Origin: United States, Selected Years 1950–2018." In *Health, United States, 2019*. Hyattsville, MD: National Center for Health Statistics, 2021. https://www.cdc.gov/nchs/data/hus/2019/005-508.pdf.

"NCHS—Infant Mortality Rates by Race: United States, 1915–2013." Centers for Disease Control and Prevention, June 5, 2020. https://data.cdc.gov/NCHS/NCHS-Infant-Mortality-Rates-by-Race-United-States-/ddsk-zebd.

Nicholls, Keith. "Politics and Civil Rights in Post–World War II Mobile." In Thomason, *Mobile*, 247–76.

Nixon, Richard M. "Special Message to the Congress Proposing a National Health Strategy." February 18, 1971. American Presidency Project, US Santa Barbara, accessed July 13, 2023. https://www.presidency.ucsb.edu/documents/special-message-the-congress-proposing-national-health-strategy.

Numbers, Ronald. *Almost Persuaded: American Physicians and Compulsory Health Insurance, 1912–1920*. Baltimore, MD: Johns Hopkins Press, 1978.

Obama, Barack. *A Promised Land*. New York: Crown, 2020.

Oberlander, Jonathan, and Theodore R. Marmor. "The Road Not Taken: What Happened to Medicare for All?" In *Medicare and Medicaid at 50: America's Entitlement Programs in the Age of Affordable Care*, edited by Alan B. Cohen, David C. Colby, Keith A. Wailoo, and Julian E. Zelizer, 55–74. New York: Oxford University Press, 2015.

Oldstone, Michael B. A. *Viruses, Plagues, and History*. New York: Oxford University Press, 2020.

Pauly, Mark V., Patricia Damon, Paul Feldstein, and John Hoff. "A Plan for 'Responsible National Health Insurance.'" *Health Affairs* 10, no. 1 (Spring 1991): 5–25. https://doi.org/10.1377/hlthaff.10.1.5.

Peters, Jeremy W. "*Sarah Palin v. New York Times* Spotlights Push to Loosen Libel Law." *New York Times*, January 23, 2022, https://www.nytimes.com/2022/01/23/business/media/sarah-palin-libel-suit-nyt.html.

Pierson, Paul. "Path Dependence, Increasing Returns, and the Study of Politics." *American Political Science Review* 33, no. 6/7 (2000): 251–67.

Poen, Monte M. *Harry S. Truman versus the Medical Lobby*. Columbia: University of Missouri Press, 1979.

Pride, Richard A. *The Confession of Dorothy Danner*. Nashville, TN: Vanderbilt University Press, 1995.

———. *The Political Use of Racial Narratives: School Desegregation in Mobile, Alabama, 1954–97*. Urbana: University of Illinois Press, 2002.

Quadagno, Jill. *The Color of Welfare: How Racism Undermined the War on Poverty*. Oxford: Oxford University Press, 1994.

Reagan, Ronald. "Inaugural Address 1981," January 20, 1981. Ronald Reagan Presidential Library and Museum, accessed July 13, 2023. https://www.reaganlibrary.gov/archives/speech/inaugural-address-1981.

Redford, Gabrielle. "AAMC Renames Prestigious Abraham Flexner Award in Light of Racist and Sexist Writings." Association of American Medical Colleges, Nov. 17, 2020, https://www.aamc.org/news-insights/aamc-renames-prestigious-abraham-flexner-award-light-racist-and-sexist-writings.

Relman, Arnold S. "The New Medical-Industrial Complex." *New England Journal of Medicine* 303, no. 11 (1980): 963–70.

Renschler, Emily S., and Janet Monge. 2008. "The Samuel George Morton Cranial Collection." *Expedition* 50, no. 3 (2008): 30–38.

Richardson, Fredrick Douglas, Jr. *The Genesis and Exodus of NOW*, 2nd ed. Self-published. CreateSpace, 2014.

Robertson, Campbell. "Alabama Simmers Before Vote on Its Constitution's Racist Language." *New York Times*, October 32, 2012. https://www.nytimes.com/2012/10/31/us/alabama-simmers-before-vote-on-its-constitutions-racist-language.html

Robertson, Natalie S. *The Slave Ship* Clotilda *and the Making of AfricaTown, USA*. Westport, CT: Praeger, 2008.

Roche, Roberta Senechal de la. *In Lincoln's Shadow: The 1908 Race Riot in Springfield, Illinois*. Carbondale: Southern Illinois University Press, 2008.

Rogers, William Warren, Robert David Ward, Leah Rawls Atkins, and Wayne Flynt. *Alabama: The History of a Deep South State*. Tuscaloosa: University of Alabama Press, 1994.

Rosenthal, Caitlin. "Slavery's Scientific Management: Masters and Managers." In *Slavery's Capitalism*, edited by Sven Beckert and Seth Rockham, 62–86. Philadelphia: University of Pennsylvania Press, 2016.

Rothstein, Richard. *The Color of Law: A Forgotten History of How Our Government Segregated America*. New York: Liveright, 2017.

Roy, Avik. "The Tortuous History of Conservatives and the Individual Mandate." *Forbes*, February 7, 2012.

Salisbury, Stephan. "Origins of Skulls Held by Penn Hard to Untangle." *Philadelphia Inquirer*, February 16, 2021. https://www.inquirer.com/news/penn-museum-morton-collection-black-philadelphians-skulls-20210216.html.

Scarupa, Harriet J. "W. Montague Cobb: His Long, Storied, Battle-Scarred Life." *New Directions* 15, no. 2 (1988). https://dh.howard.edu/newdirections/vol15/iss2/2.

Schneider, Eric C., Arnav Shah, Michelle M. Doty, Roosa Tikkanen, Katharine Fields, and Reginald D. Williams II. "Mirror, Mirror 2021—Reflecting Poorly: Health Care in the U.S. Compared to Other High-Income Countries." Fund Reports, The Commonwealth Fund, August 4, 2021. https://www.commonwealthfund.org/publications/fund-reports/2021/aug/mirror-mirror-2021-reflecting-poorly.

Schulman, Kevin A., Jesse A. Berlin, William Harless, et al. "The Effect of Race and Sex on Physicians' Recommendations for Cardiac Catheterization." *New England Journal of Medicine* 340, no. 8 (1999): 618–26.

Scribner, Christopher MacGregor. "Progress versus Tradition in Mobile, 1900–1920." In Thomason, *Mobile*.

Segal, Ronald. *The Black Diaspora: Five Centuries of the Black Experience Outside Africa*. New York: Farrar, Straus and Giroux, 1995.

Sister Maria. "History of St. Martin de Porres Hospital, Mobile, Alabama." *Journal of the National Medical Association* 56, no. 4 (1964): 303–6.

Skloot, Rebecca. *The Immortal Life of Henrietta Lacks*. New York: Random House, 2011.

Skowronek, Stephen. "The Reassociation of Ideas and Purposes: Racism, Liberalism, and the American Political Tradition." *American Political Science Review* 100, no. 3 (2006): 385–401.

Smith, David Barton. "Addressing Racial Inequities in Health Care: Civil Rights Monitoring and Report Cards." *Journal of Health Politics, Policy and Law* 23, no. 1 (1998): 75–105. https://doi.org/10.1215/03616878-23-1-75.

———. "Forgotten Heroes: Remembering Dr. Alvin Blount, Who Helped Integrate America's Hospitals." *Health Affairs Blog*, September 1, 2017. https://www.healthaffairs.org/do/10.1377/hblog20170901.061774/full.

———. *Health Care Divided: Race and Healing a Nation*. Ann Arbor: University of Michigan Press, 1999.

———. "Jim Crow Medicine and the Elusive Pursuit of Universal Care." In *The Oxford Handbook of American Medical History*, edited by James A. Schafer Jr., Richard M. Mizelle, and Helen K. Valier. New York: Oxford University Press, in press.

———. "The Pandemic Challenge: End Separate and Unequal Healthcare." *American Journal of Medical Sciences* 360, no. 2 (2020): 109–11. https://doi.org/10.1016%2Fj.amjms.2020.04.011.

———. "The Politics of Racial Disparities: Desegregating the Hospitals in Jackson, Mississippi." *Milbank Quarterly* 83, no. 5 (2005): 247–69. https://doi.org/10.1111%2Fj.1468-0009.2005.00346.x.

———. "Population Ecology and the Racial Integration of Hospitals and Nursing Homes in the United States." *Milbank Quarterly* 68, no. 4 (1990): 561–96. https://doi.org/10.2307/3350194.

———. *The Power to Heal: Civil Rights, Medicare, and the Struggle to Transform America's Health Care System*. Nashville, TN: Vanderbilt University Press, 2016.

———. "The Racial Segregation of Hospital Care Revisited: Medicare Discharge Patterns and Their Implications." *American Journal of Public Health* 88, no. 3 (1998): 461–63. https://doi.org/10.2105/AJPH.88.3.461.

Smith, David Barton, Zhanlian Feng, Mary L. Fennell, Jacqueline Zinn, and Vincent Mor. "Racial Disparities in Access to Long-Term Care: The Illusive Pursuit of Equity." *Journal of Health Politics, Policy and Law* 33, no. 5 (2008): 861–81. https://doi.org/10.1215/03616878-2008-022.

———. "Separate and Unequal: Racial Segregation and Disparities in Quality Across U.S. Nursing Homes." *Health Affairs* 26, no. 5 (2007): 1448–58. https://doi.org/10.1377/hlthaff.26.5.1448.

Smith, John David, and J. Vincent Lowery, eds. *The Dunning School.* Lexington: University Press of Kentucky, 2013.

Snowden, Frank M. *Epidemics and Society: From the Black Death to the Present.* New Haven, CT: Yale University Press, 2020.

Southern, David W. *The Malignant Heritage: Yankee Progressives and the Negro Question, 1901–1914.* Chicago: Loyola University Press, 1968.

Staples, Brent. "The Burning of Black Wall Street, Revisited." *New York Times,* June 19, 2020. https://www.nytimes.com/2020/06/19/opinion/tulsa-race-riot-massacre-graves.html.

Starr, Paul. *The Social Transformation of American Medicine.* New York: Harper Collins, 1982.

Stevenson, Robert Lewis. *The Strange Case of Dr. Jekyll and Mr. Hyde.* London: Longmans, Green and Company, 1886.

Stone, Deborah. "The Struggle for the Soul of Health Insurance." *Journal of Health Politics, Policy and Law* 18, no. 2 (1993): 287–317.

Swarns, Rachel L. "272 Slaves Were Sold to Save Georgetown. What Does It Owe Their Descendants?" *New York Times,* April 16, 2016. www.nytimes.com/2016/04/17/us/georgetown-university-search-for-slave-descendents.html.

———. "Insurance Policies on Slaves: New York Life's Complicated Past." *New York Times,* December 18, 2016. http://www.nytimes.com/2016/12/18/us/insurance-policies-on-slaves-new-york-lifes-complicated-past.html.

Tarbert, Jesse. *When Good Government Meant Big Government: The Quest to Expand Federal Power, 1913–1933.* New York: Columbia University Press, 2022.

Thomas, Karen Kruse. *Deluxe Jim Crow: Civil Rights and American Health Policy, 1935–1954.* Athens: University of Georgia Press, 2011.

Thomason, Michael V. R., ed. *Mobile: The New History of Alabama's First City.* Tuscaloosa: University of Alabama Press, 2001.

Tikkanen, Roosa. "Multinational Comparisons of Health Systems Data, 2017." Commonwealth Fund, November 15, 2017. https://doi.org/10.26099/y2kb-sx06.

Tomlinson, Brett, and Carlett Spike. "Princeton Renames Wilson School and Residential College, Citing Former President's Racism." *Princeton Alumni Weekly,* June 27, 2020. https://paw.princeton.edu/print/232221.

Toobin, Jeffrey. "Keeping Speech Robust and Free." *New York Review of Books,* July 20, 2023: 27-29. https://www.nybooks.com/articles/2023/07/20/keeping-speech-robust-and-free-new-york-times-v-sullivan.

Totenberg, Nina. "Supreme Court Unexpectedly Upholds Provision Prohibiting Racial Gerrymandering." National Public Radio, June 8, 2023. https://www.npr.org/2023/06/08/1181002182/supreme-court-voting-rights.

Troller-Renfree, Sonya V., Molly A. Costanzo, Greg J. Duncan, et al. "The Impact of a Poverty Reduction Intervention on Infant Brain Activity." *Proceedings of the National Academy of Sciences* 119, no. 5 (2002): 1–8.

Truman, Harry S. "Special Message to Congress Recommending a Comprehensive Health Program." In *Public Papers of the Presidents of the United States: Harry S. Truman, 1945–1953*. Washington, DC: US Government Printing Office, 1966.

United Nations System Task Team on the Post-2015 UN Development Agenda. 2012. "Health in the Post-2015 UN Development Agenda: Thematic Think Piece." World Health Organization, May 2012, https://www.un.org/millenniumgoals/pdf/Think%20Pieces/8_health.pdf.

United States Department of Justice. "The Attorney General's Ninth Annual Report to Congress Pursuant to the Emmett Till Unsolved Civil Rights Crime Act of 2007 and Third Annual Report to Congress Pursuant to the Emmett Till Unsolved Civil Rights Crimes Reauthorization Act of 2016." March 1, 2021. https://www.justice.gov/crt/file/1405431/download.

———. "The Attorney General's Second Annual Report to Congress Pursuant to the Emmett Till Unsolved Civil Rights Crime Act of 2007." May 13, 2010. https://www.justice.gov/sites/default/files/crt/legacy/2015/06/18/tillreport_02.pdf.

Verney, Kevern. "'Every Man Should Try': John L. LeFlore and the National Association for the Advancement of Colored People in Alabama, 1919–1956." *Alabama Review* 66, no. 3 (2013): 186–210. https://doi.org/10.1353/ala.2013.0018.

Villarreal, Daniel. "69 Percent of Americans Want Medicare for All, including 46 Percent of Republicans, New Poll Says." *Newsweek*, April 24, 2020. https://www.newsweek.com/69-percent-americans-want-medicare-all-including-46-percent-republicans-new-poll-says-1500187.

Waite, Frederick C. "Grave Robbing in New England." *Bulletin of the Medical Library Association* 33 (1945): 272–94.

Walker, Samuel. *Presidents and Civil Liberties from Wilson to Obama: A Story of Poor Custodians*. New York: Cambridge University Press, 2012.

Whitmire, Kyle. "State of Denial: How 155 Angry White Men Chained Alabama to Its Confederate Past," AL.com, December 5, 2022. https://www.al.com/news/2022/12/the-curse-of-1901-how-155-angry-white-men-chained-alabama-to-its-confederate-past.html.

Wilder, Craig Steven. *Ebony and Ivy: Race, Slavery, and the Troubled History of America's Universities*. New York: Bloomsbury Press, 2013.

Wilkerson, Isabel. *Caste: The Origins of Our Discontents*. New York: Random House, 2020.

Wilson, Kenneth L., Wayne L. DeBeatham, Omar K. Danner, L. Ray Matthew, Louise N. Bacon, and William Lynn Weaver. "The Forgotten MASH Surgeon: The Story of Alvin Vincent Blount Jr, MD." *Journal of the National Medical Association* 104, no. 3 (2012): 221–23.

Wilson, Woodrow. *A History of the American People*. New York: Harper, 1917.

Woodward, C. Vann. *The Strange Career of Jim Crow*. New York: Oxford University Press, 1955.

World Health Organization. "Universal Health Coverage." Accessed May 25, 2023. https://www.who.int/news-room/fact-sheets/detail/universal-health-coverage-(uhc).

Yellin, Eric S. *Racism in the Nation's Service: Government Workers and the Color Line in Woodrow Wilson's America*. Chapel Hill: University of North Carolina Press, 2013.

Zinn, Howard. *You Can't Be Neutral on a Moving Train*. Boston, MA: Beacon Press, 1995.

Zucchino, David. *Wilmington's Lie: The Murderous Coup of 1898 and the Rise of White Supremacy*. New York: Atlantic Monthly Press, 2020.

INDEX

Page numbers in *italic* refer to figures and tables.

ACKNOWLEDGMENTS

IT TOOK MORE THAN THIRTY YEARS to pull this book together. The list of those I am indebted for help grew. I hope in this brief outline that those not specifically mentioned by name will recognize the part that they played and accept my acknowledgment as well.

Colleagues at the two academic institutions I have been most recently connected to, Temple and Drexel University, gave permission and encouragement. In Temple's Health Management and Policy group I would especially like to thank Bill Aaronson, Stuart Fine, Tom Getzen, Chuck Hall (deceased), and Jackline Zinn for their suggestions and encouragement. The Health Management and Policy Department in the Dornsife School of Public Health of Drexel University has placed a special emphasis on social justice. Colleagues Daryl Brown, James Buehler, Robert Field, Marla Gold, and Alex Ortega have been important resources and sources of encouragement in completing this book. Jan Eberth, Drexel's chair of the Department of Health Management and Policy has been particularly helpful and encouraging of this effort. Students in both these programs have provided much stimulation and many insights.

Many "real world" experiences, working with those outside universities contributed as well. Early in my career I served as an Intergovernmental Personnel Act (IPA) Fellow with the Office of Research and Policy in what has since become The Center for Medicare and

Medicaid Services (CMS) in the Department of Health and Human Services (DHHS) in Washington, DC. I also assisted more than twenty different hospital systems with conducting community health needs assessments. In addition, I served as an evaluator of a Commonwealth Fund national demonstration project overseen by Mary Jane Koren, MD, that engaged in quality improvement in poorly performing nursing homes serving majority Black populations. Most recently during the COVID pandemic, I served on an advisory committee that helped create a health department in Delaware County, Pennsylvania. These experiences shaped the story told in this book. I am indebted to the many fine people I had the opportunity to work and learn from.

An old family friend, Walter Adams, revered economics professor and, briefly, president of Michigan State University, once advised me that if you really want to learn how the "system" works, sue it. It proved a remarkable insight but not something by temperament or resources I could ever imagine doing. Some talented lawyers committed to social justice did sue and allowed me to assist as an expert witness. The first suit, *Taylor v. White*, No. 90–3307 (E. D. an amended complaint filed August 15, 1990) involved the failure of the Secretary of Welfare of the state of Pennsylvania to enforce compliance of Title VI of the Civil Rights Act in assuring equitable access to nursing homes for Black elders. As an expert witness it was an easy case to make with statistics. The Pennsylvania Health Law Project brought the suit. Ann Torregrossa, Michael Campbell, and Phillip Tannenbaum did the legal work on the case. The second suit was brought against the secretary of the Department of Health and Human Services for failure to collect any data or do any analysis to determine whether providers receiving Medicare and Medicaid funding followed Title VI (*Madison-Hughes v. Shalala*, No. 3–93–0046 [M.D. Tenn., filed January 19, 1993]). As an expert witness, it was even an easier case. HHS had done nothing to ascertain compliance and all I had to do was say that the Emperor (or Empress in this case, since the defendant was Secretary Donna Shalala) had no clothes. Gordon Bonnyman of the Tennessee Justice Center and others connected to the Poverty and Race Research Action Council (PRRAC) brought the suit. Those bringing both suits were exceptionally talented and committed and I learned a great deal from their efforts. Neither suit was successful. A summary of the details are provided elsewhere.[1] I had, indeed, learned a lot about how the "system" works.[2] It does not. That meant either devoting more effort to understanding how to change it or to just disengage.

That decision was made for me when I was awarded a Robert Wood Johnson (RWJ) Health Policy Investigator Award in 1994. I had the time and travel resources to capture some of the story, but time was running out. Those directly involved in the key health care civil rights efforts in the 1930s to the 1960s were dying off. They were an amazing courageous group with wonderful insights and untold stories.

The RWJ project produced *Health Care Divided*, a book that captured the interest of Barbara Berney in creating a documentary film.[3] Our plan was to focus on the critical six-month period prior to the implementation of the Medicare program and release both a book and documentary in July 2016 for the fiftieth anniversary of Medicare's implementation. The book met that deadline but the documentary, a far more complicated process, took another two years.[4] Charles Burnett and David Lowenthal, both with distinguished film careers, served as directors. Barbara Burney served as producer. Danny Glover, more of an art film intellectual and activist than the buddy-cop action film hero he is most known for, served as the narrator. It has been aired on many PBS stations, viewed at universities by undergraduates, medical, and allied health students, and by community groups. Both Barbara and I have served as commentators at many of these events. I am indebted to Barbara's persistence, for the additional resources she provided through interviews and documentation, and for all the exciting presentations which the film produced.

There was only one final layer of the larger story left undone: trying to make sense of the death of Jean Cowsert, MD, and how that death might be linked to the nation's unchanging health disparities and the failure to assure universal access to health care. For this, I needed help. I knew nothing about how to investigate a cold case nor had any familiarity with the community where the events took place.

Early interviews in Mobile, Alabama with those also fascinated with its medical history hooked me. They were all fascinating storytellers. I am particularly indebted to Sam Eichold, MD, custodian of Mobile's medical history for his insights. Also to Joy H. P. Harriman, who as medical librarian at the Mobile Infirmary had the opportunity to interview many of the physicians and other health professionals connected to that institution. She produced an oral history of those familiar with Mobile medical history in the 1940s and '50s.[5] That collection and her help in understanding all the hospital-social dynamics of Mobile were invaluable. Natives of Mobile and professional historians Frye Gaillard and Scotty Kirkland were key resources. Gaillard is an inspiring master storyteller about the civil rights struggles in Alabama.[6] Kirkland has focused on the less accessible but fascinating civil rights story of Mobile, Alabama.

Many individuals connected to the University of Alabama in Birmingham, Jean Cowsert's medical school alma mater) were encouraging and supportive. Two individuals went out of their way to be helpful to this effort. Christy Lemak, professor and former longtime chair of the deservedly top ranked Department of Health Services Management, was invaluable in encouraging this project and connecting me with key resources at the University and hospitals in Alabama. Richard deShazo, MD, a native of Birmingham, former chair of medicine at the University of Southern Alabama in Mobile, chair of medicine at the University of Mississippi in Jackson, and now back in Birmingham at the University of Alabama's medical school was an invaluable resource. Dr. deShazo provided many insights into medicine in Mobile and in Alabama. He published an invaluable resource into the history of civil rights in medicine in the South.[7] He also facilitated in the publication of a commentary based on one of the chapters in this book in a key medical journal.[8] Most importantly, he waded through several poorly written and organized drafts of this book, without giving up, making corrective suggestions. I am most grateful for his help.

Left undone was help in investigating a civil rights cold case. I was most fortunate to enlist the assistance of Margaret Burnham, a native of Birmingham, civil rights lawyer, judge and then professor at Northeastern University School of Law. She helped create at Northeastern the Civil Rights Restorative Justice Project (CRRJ), to attempt to address the gap between the family disappointment produced by mostly unsuccessful federal prosecution of Jim Crow Era race related murders. Families of victims, at the very least, needed as best that could be determined the facts surrounding the death and some formal acknowledgment in terms of ceremony, apology, or physical marker of the event. A database of more than one thousand cases now exists as a resource for families and researchers. A half dozen of these cases related to Mobile are included in this book. Burnham has also used them in a beautifully written, powerful book offering new insights into the Jim Crow Era.[9] Rose Zoltek-Jick, who serves as associate director of the project, was more than generous in answering my many questions, recruiting student to assist, and helping to provide access to the CCRJ project database. I am particularly indebted to the three talented students who were assigned to the Jean Cowsert case, Fraser Grier, Noah Lapidus, and Seth Reiner.

They helped flesh out the story further and rework it in legal language that helped bring the case to the attention of the Emmett Till Cold Case Investigation team in the Justice Department. In 2022 the Justice Department and the FBI opened an Emmett Till Cold Case Investigation into Jean Cowsert's death. It is one of twenty-five cases still open on a list that includes 161. An FBI agent in their Mobile office and civil rights lawyer in the Justice Department head the investigation. Dr. Cowsert's surviving family members are delighted by the attention provided by investigators. She is the only physician on the list and only white person among the open cases. I was also delighted in that the DOJ's involvement assures a careful, thorough, and professional investigation and an opportunity to give her some of the long-delayed recognition she deserves.

None of this would have been possible without the patience and encouragement of key people at Vanderbilt Press. Zachary Gresham helped provide the initial encouragement for completing this project and guiding me through the review process. Gianna Mosser helped with encouragement and smoothing the rough patches in the production process. Betsy Phillips helped with the books marketing abetted by her own interests in the more sinister sides of the Civil Rights Era. Joell Smith-Borne, whose help with an earlier book sold me on Vanderbilt, did the magic and hard work in the editing and production process. Lisa DeBoer completed the final job of indexing masterfully under a tight deadline. Thanks to all of you and all the others that chipped in.

Family and friends were not spared from the obsession related to completing this book. As always my wife, Joan Apt, assisted with careful editing. Longtime friend Bob Uris sharpened his editing skills as a former newspaper reporter on early drafts. My sister, Barbara Smith, a professional writer, and former civil rights activist during the 1960s did a thorough editing of an early version of the entire manuscript.

The final product is my own. Unfortunately, too often remotely during the COVID pandemic, it has been wonderful to have such helpful and interesting people to exchange ideas. Their contributions made this book possible and account for its strengths.

Printed in the USA
CPSIA information can be obtained
at www.ICGtesting.com
LVHW051326041023
760025LV00004B/252